SHuzie: A m

My Journey of Lung Cancer to Brain Metastasis

Preface

I wrapped my puny arms around her prickly middle and gently moved forward for a kiss. She was like a gorilla and I a small child as I struggled to touch her strength. Moving forward, I took a deep breath in and smelled the essence of her flowery and woody flavor that stuck to the insides of my nose while it lasted.

"Thank you, Shuzie." I took another sweet breath in and held it. As my face departed our moment I ran my right hand over the fluffy pink flowers like cotton candy sitting on the twigs waiting for someone to abscond them.

I look around suspiciously. Had anyone seen me? That could be embarrassing, I thought to myself. I mean, really. Hugging and kissing a tree? Who does that? I shook my head and smiled to myself. Okay, I am known to be a little dorky from time to time…this being one of those times! But the coast was clear. No one had seen me. At least not my neighbors.

I loved the intricate beauty of trees since I can remember. The sway of the willows; the strength of the oak; the beauty of flowering crabapple trees. I drew their delicate twigs over and over on paper like an obsession. Now every year my husband would take me out for Mother's Day and let me pick out my own personal tree and I would name it.

I told myself that if Shuzie could anchor herself against a blustery, cold Maine wind than I could withstand cancer. That's what she whispered in my ear, anyway. I decided, in that moment, to be strong; to be the center of attention although it made me uncomfortable. I would bend; but not break (quoting lyrics from the singer, Pink).

Shuzie was a mother's day gift from my husband a couple of years ago. Ever since, she has blossomed into a gorgeous pink and purple crabapple tree. She produces crabapples but they can't be eaten. They look like dark purple plump raisins, but it's all a façade. It's more proof from her that she can do it; if she wanted. I ate one once and was never able to swallow the contents.

Why Shuzie, you ask? I took the first couple letters of my name and the last few letters of my mother-in-laws name to come up with Shuzie – a combination of Sherry and my mother-in-laws nick name, Suzie. The sound was like a whispering when the wind tunneled through the flowers.

I felt the homage to be appropriate since Susan died at the tender age of fifty-five from Parkinson's disease. For some reason, I always felt Susan was here...close by...in that tree – watching and whispering her guarded knowledge.

Chapter 1

Pain in the Neck

I tossed my black leather bag into my locker and gave a quick glance in the mirror for any straggler's. My hand reached for the left side of my scrubs pocket and I felt my lip gloss; the right side proved to contain my neat row of black and blue pens with the covers attached to my black pants (yes, I am a dork).

I reached for the door and headed for the coffee station, ever sure to take a peek into each room along the way to see what I was in for during my shift. It shouldn't be too bad, I thought to myself, it was January 6th and people were probably still in the holiday spirit.

The other technician welcomed my arrival and I smiled for feeling needed. As he gave me a brief report regarding each room, I lost focus and turned in my chair to see the doctors who were scheduled during my shift. Who was scheduled told me how well or how quickly the shift would be run.

Back to my technician report and with a happy sigh I finished the report and thanked my colleague. "Oh, and you might hear screaming." Said my partner. "Oh, great." I said smiling sarcastically. I was used to the screaming, yelling and hostility from some of the emergency room clients. That never bothered me. The thing that made up for it was the good people I was able to help.

Even the screaming banshees needed something or someone. So I snickered when I was asked to help the gentleman - who was not such a gentleman - as everyone had grown tired of him by eleven in the morning. I had a knack at accommodating the worst – drug abusers, Alzheimer's patients, teen-agers and even the kind like my gentleman in room five. It was time to find out what I could do for him.

I said my 'hellos' to everyone along the way and knocked on the door. Someone had his door ajar in a feeble attempt to try stifling his swearing. But before I made my way in, someone whispered to be careful, for he was known to spit. I nodded, not surprised by the exchange.

"Well, hello." I said confidently. "How are you?" I headed over to the gloved area as I eyed his physique. He was grossly dirty with overgrown hair and long yellow fingernails. I smiled at him anyway.

"Roger (not his real name), I'm Sherry. I'm here to help you. What can I get for you?" As I snapped a grey glove on. "Oh, Sherry. It's so nice to meet you." He said in his most pleasant voice. I cocked my head to the side and said, "Wow Roger, you have a reputation around here but you sure seem nice enough to me." We both laughed.

Once I said that, we were friends. He asked if I could pour him some water, give him the television remote and put the phone next to him in bed. Mostly, he just wanted to vent. I did everything possible to accommodate him. As I was leaving the room, he whined, "Sherry, one more thing. Could you adjust me up in bed?"

"Of course." I said. I went to the back of his bed and he grabbed the rails. "Ready?" I said as I grabbed the sheet behind him. "One, two, three." I yelled and pulled up on the white sheet. Immediately, I felt a pull on the left side of my back.

Looking down, I finally realized that my patient had no feet and had not helped in pulling himself upward. I mentally kicked myself. I knew better. I remember an instructor once telling me in C.N.A. class that a career is not worth the person and to be careful with back injuries for it can ruin a career.

I graduated the top of my class in Augusta and should have known better so I said nothing. I left the room and kept reliving the moment as the ache in my back throbbed on my left shoulder. People asked what was wrong, but I downplayed it. I thought for sure it would go away the next day.

The next day after the next, the pain didn't go away. It spread. What had started in my scapula, eventually traveled up my spine, down my left shoulder and arm and ended with numbness in two of my fingers.

At this point, I had used heat warmers, ice packs, massage, relaxation and hot showers to no avail.

After ten days of grumbling, my friend Donna suggested that I see a chiropractor. I didn't even know a chiropractor. I opened up the yellow pages and reluctantly, I called. I was given an appointment the next day, a few minutes from my house.

Chapter 2

Funny Bones

I pulled the scarf up past my nose and walked briskly but carefully over the crunch of the ice and to the chiropractor's office. I was their first appointment of the day and got there early to ensure a parking space. I tried to smile through the pain to make idle chit-chat with the receptionist while I waited. But even Enya playing over the speakers couldn't slow down my heart.

Finally, by the time Dr. Blaine Curtis came into the room, he could see I was in obvious pain. He was pleasant, asked me to sit down and immediately began to check the adjustments in my neck and spine. After he was satisfied with his work, he said, "I do believe you have either a bulging or herniated disc. I am going to recommend to your primary care provider that you should have this looked at."

I groaned. He continued, "In the meantime, I am going to set you up with electrode therapy which may help some of the muscles that are involved." I eavesdropped on the conversation as he spoke with my primary care provider. Always the procrastinator, I thought about making the provider switch now that I actually had a problem going on.

While I laid on the table, I thought about who I was going to change my primary care provider to and made up my mind on a hospitalist who works in the same hospital as me. After I got home, I called the emergency room and spoke to a physician who said I should come in and that the MRI folks were fortunately still working after five at night and could scan my head. I threw all caution to the wind and went.

After multiple tests, including blood work, an

EKG and a routine work up, I was sent to have my first

MRI. I quietly thanked God as the MRI people would

not normally be ready and able to scan me but they

happened to be there after hours, according to my

emergency room physician, Dr. James Kilgour.

However, I was still scared as hell.

I was asked to change my clothing, take off my

jewelry and lie on a metal table. After I chose classical

music to listen to, I was stuffed backwards into the easy

bake MRI where I cooked for twenty five minutes

while I tried not to panic that I was in an enclosed

space. "Don't look." I'd tell myself. "Don't open your

eyes."

I meditated to the music and refused to open my

eyes to see that I was seemingly lying in my own

casket. I actually began to feel so relaxed that I fell

asleep for a few moments. My body shook myself out of my slumber and I opened my eyes. My dumbfounded eyes. Why did I do that? I looked like an English guardsman for the remainder of my ride.

The physician came in after a short while and confirmed a bulging and a herniated disk and disk fragments around Cervical 5-Cervical 7, in my neck. If that wasn't scary enough, the doctor said, "Also, as an insignificant finding, we found something growing in your brain." He paused. "It appears benign." I exhaled. "It's probably been there since birth." He studied me.

I breathed through the rest and looked at my husband who wasn't paying attention to what was being said, as there was a child and a lot of activity in the room. I confirmed, "Ok, so this growth is nothing to worry about." The physician confirmed that and said he spoke with the radiologist and they were both in agreement.

To be sure, he gave me a short neurological exam, which I passed. Dr. Kilgour suggested that I use traction for my neck and to take the prescribed medications. He also had me follow-up with a neurologist in the same hospital for later on that week.

It was a quiet ride home. I finally broke the silence. "David, did you hear what the doctor said about my head?" He looked surprised and said, "No." I said, "Okay, so I shouldn't worry then that they found something growing in my brain that appears benign since birth?" He was shocked and hadn't heard any of that conversation. Well, I told myself, if it were important, David would have heard it. I'm sure it was nothing. I thought nothing more of it.

Chapter 3

If I Only Had a Brain

I had just spooned some mint chocolate chip ice cream into a dish and sat down on my favorite sofa with my favorite blankey in my favorite feline position on the couch when....rrrriiinnnggg. My body shook in tune with the phone. It jarred my peace and tranquility. I breathed deeply to slow down my heart and slowly moved toward the receiver. Judge Mathis would have to wait.

"Hello?" I asked. "Sherry, its Kenzie." I knew immediately from her childlike voice that it was McKenzie Savidge, or Dr. Savidge, an Emergency Room Doctor. My guard flew up. "Hey, what's up,

Kenzie?" I imagined her bouncing in her seat, eating left over Thai food.

"Remember that MRI you had yesterday?" My chest started to feel heavy. "Yes?" She swallowed. "After the doc and the radiologist looked at it last night, a second radiologist looked at it. It looks like he's ordering a Brain MRI with contrast. He wants a better look at the image. If you want to schedule that for next week, that's fine."

"Oh, okay." Guess what? Not okay! I worried for a week what this meant. On one hand I was scared to death; on the other hand I thought if it were really serious, then my MRI would be scheduled for the next day. However, it was the following week on 1/24/13 that I was scheduled for the brain MRI with contrast.

For those of you who have never had an MRI (like myself), let me explain the process to you, in detail.

If you haven't died yet, this will make you believe that you have! I was asked to change my clothes into the glorious hospital garb and remove my jewelry. I had a nose ring and a belly button ring which I couldn't remove. The MRI tech said it may burn my skin or give false results. That was too bad…'cause it wasn't coming out! It didn't come out the first time and it wasn't coming out the second time.

He reviewed a million different questions (okay, I'm exaggerating!), then said, "Do you have a hundred and fifty dollars today?" I balked. "How much is the MRI?" The technician guessed it to be a little under $2,000. The insurance company probably wanted me to pay because it was an incidental finding. Well, guess what? We were minus in our bank account balance at the time and I sure as hell wasn't going to go without an MRI to see if I had a brain tumor! It was not an incidental finding to me.

I looked him in the eye and said, "No, I don't have the money." And sat stoically. There was silence, then he said, "Okay. I guess you can work that out with the insurance company."

I stepped up the stairs of the frigid trailer and followed my tech to a small room with a huge casket-like MRI scanner. He asked me to get onto the MRI bench. "What kind of music do you like?" Really, I thought, sarcastically. This is not Match.com.

I looked at him with suspicion then realized he meant what kind of music I would like to listen to while being scanned. I told him classical – especially under the circumstances. He smiled and put headphones on me. Okay; I was a little uptight – but for good reason.

"How long do you think this test will take?" I asked while taking off my shoes. "About twenty minutes." He said. "In the middle of the test we'll give you a shot of contrast. Have a seat."

I mustered the courage to maintain my dignity while I tugged at my hospital gown which emphatically refused to go my way while I tried to lie down. I made the decision again that I would close my eyes and not look. That was a good choice because a few seconds later he put down a mask a few inches from my face and pushed the button to move me backward into the dark tunnel. Hello, claustrophobia!

It was dark and it was lonely – a weird description but that's what it felt like to me. The MRI was incredibly noisy and pounded in my ears in the forefront of the music. However, I focused on the classical music and never opened my eyes. I stayed completely still to ensure I didn't have to do the test again.   Funny the things that you think of when everything else has cleared from your mind.

I remember intuitively thinking that it would be funny – but not ha, ha funny – if the radiologist found something else in this MRI besides the neck issues. Finally, I heard a voice in my earphones after a few minutes of contrast that we were done.   It was the technician.   I could have clapped!   But that would be…Sherry, I guess! The same Sherry who would hum the tune, "If I Only Had a Brain", during work and hoped no one would take offense to it, not six months before I was diagnosed. If only I knew then, what I know now.

Chapter 4

Houston…We Have a Problem

On 1/25/13, I scheduled an appointment to meet with my new primary care provider, Dr. Kevin Davey. I reviewed my story with him. He had me perform a neurological exam. I should have brought a video camera because surely I would have won America's Funniest Home Videos. Picture me hopping on one foot, tapping my nose, walking on my heels and my toes. I kept thinking he was going to pull out a Breathalyzer!

After the neurological exam was completed, we both sat down. He said he thought that this lesion in my brain had been there since birth and we would keep an eye on it. I silently agreed since I was passing all the neurological exams. I was satisfied and relieved with his response, for now. However, I had a pit in my stomach about the future.

I assured my primary care provider that I would keep him posted about my neurological appointment the next day. The purpose of the exam was to review cervical bones five through seven in my neck and to briefly review the incidental finding of the lesion in my brain with the neurologist. I expected an in and out appointment, so I took my son, Joseph, with me.

At a year and a half, Joseph was a mischievous handful. I say he is pure genius and that's probably because I'm his mother! But also because he has the personality of Curious George. The appointment was mid-morning and I was anxious to get it over with and to get Joseph home for a nap. We named him Joseph Kenneth because his first name is David's father and the middle name is my father's. Not sure it was the best combo as he is full of piss and vinegar, like his ancestors!

The neurologist was a new doctor to me and I wasn't sure yet if I was going to like her. In my experience, there are doctors that have a great bedside manner but don't know that much; doctors that have a terrible bedside manner but they are great teachers and very knowledgeable; and those who come right down the middle like Plinko.

I would rather have a doctor with a compassionate bedside manner who loves to teach their craft. Unfortunately, the doctor I was sent to was not a good fit with me.

As Joe bounced on my lap and attempted to five finger discount everything on her desk, the doctor explained that I indeed herniated one disc, bulged another and that there were disc fragments next to my spine. She didn't seemed concerned about this and stated that the fragments would simply dissolve into my body and I didn't need surgery for the herniated and bulging disk. She suggested medication and traction for the pinched nerve causing numbness down my arm into my fingers.

I was relieved. I didn't want to have spine surgery at forty-two. I was surprised the disc fragments would go away on their own. Now the real deal. What I was here for. Where was my MRI with contrast? It seemed like forever for her to pull up my records. Was she saving the best for last? There was an awkward silence in the room; only broken by the clearing of her throat.

I kissed Joe for comfort while my heart pounded out of my chest. I watched her expression as she pulled up the image on her computer. I wondered why she was so quiet. "Hmm." She said with concern. I repeated what she said in my mind. That didn't sound good.

"It looks like a slow growing cancer in your brain." I wanted to fall off the chair but I had to be strong for my son. Had I known it might be the other icky-c word – cancer - I certainly wouldn't be here with a baby on my lap on a Friday afternoon and without my husband here with me for support. "They'll definitely want to biopsy that." She said matter-of-factly.

"So, what does that entail? A needle aspiration?" It's so silly now when you think about what you said when you were in shock, isn't it? Like they could stick a needle through my skull! She said, "No. They will take out a piece of your skull. Then they'll take a piece of this lesion. Don't be surprised if they take the whole thing. Where do you want to go? Portland or Bangor?"

I swallowed hard. "Portland, I guess. We went to Maine Medical for testing when I was pregnant with Joseph." She nodded her head. "Okay. Do you want to wait in here or in the waiting room?" I looked at Joe who was running around her office now and stammered, "The waiting room."

I picked up Joe and swallowed my tears, smiling along the way, but in complete shock. I didn't want to scare Joe and I had to call my husband, David. I walked right past the patients in the waiting room and dug through my purse to find my phone. I texted David, "Houston….we have a problem."

He texted my phone several times but I didn't respond. A sweet woman in the waiting room was talking my ear off. I'm looking at her thinking, she has no idea what I have just been told. Plus, I think I needed a few moments for the word, cancer, to sink in. I nodded and shook my head as an automatic response, but had no idea what this stranger said, who was sitting beside me.

My phone rang. I looked at the number. I dreaded this phone call; and yet the person I needed most was on the other line. I picked up the phone, grabbed Joe and went into the hallway for privacy. I took a deep breath and answered the phone.

David happened to be painting right behind the hospital, just feet away from my doctor's office. He sounded frantic. I began to recite exactly what the doctor said. He kept asking me, "What does that mean?" But even I didn't know. Speaking through tears, he said he was leaving work and could be at the doctor's in a few minutes. Through broken words I told him that would be great. I couldn't wait until my husband came to make things better...but I just didn't know if he could this time.

My husband showed up a few minutes later. He just touched my face and had tears in his eyes. I swallowed hard and got up to get Joe who was now ripping the brochures into two. I seemed to do things in auto-pilot. My husband stood guard next to me. We waited in silence.

About ten minutes later, the neurologist came out holding a yellow sticky note. "Here, I'll give this to you." In cliché fashion, she handed the paper to me with a number. "It's the number of the neurosurgeon. I've been on hold all this time. They are insisting that I need to talk to the neurosurgeon and I don't. You can call the number on Monday if they don't call you." And with that, the house fell on top of her striped socks.

We stood alone in silence. Was she coming back? I guess not. What do we do now? Is it okay to leave? We looked at each other, confused.

It was Friday. Black and gloomy Friday, for me.

When I kissed David good-bye, as he was going to

follow me home with the baby, it felt different. I felt

transparent, like a ghost. His eyes were blood-shot; his

color pallor. The instant I turned on the ignition, there

was silence. Then a song came on from The Band Perry,

"If I Die Young." I didn't dare touch the radio. I just

listened to the words (the video can be found on-line):

If I die young, bury me in satin
Lay me down on a, bed of roses
Sink me in the river, at dawn
Send me away with the words of a love song
Uh oh, uh oh
Lord make me a rainbow, I'll shine down on my mother
She'll know I'm safe with you when she stands under my
colors, oh,
And life ain't always what you think it ought to be, no
Ain't even grey, but she buries her baby
The sharp knife of a short life, well
I've had just enough time
If I die young, bury me in satin
Lay me down on a bed of roses
Sink me in the river at dawn send me away with the
words of a love song
The sharp knife of a short life, well
I've had just enough time
And I'll be wearing white, when I come into your

kingdom
I'm as green as the ring on my little cold finger,
I've never known the lovin' of a man
But it sure felt nice when he was holdin' my hand,
There's a boy here in town, says he'll love me forever,
Who would have thought forever could be severed by
The sharp knife of a short life, well,
I've had just enough time
So put on your best, boys, and I'll wear my pearls
What I never did is done
A penny for my thoughts, oh, no, I'll sell 'em for a
dollar
They're worth so much more after I'm a goner
And maybe then you'll hear the words I been singin'
Funny when you're dead how people start listenin'
If I die young, bury me in satin
Lay me down on a bed of roses
Sink me in the river at dawn
Send me away with the words of a love song
Uh oh (uh, oh)
The ballad of a dove (oh, uh)
Go with peace and love
Gather up your tears, keep 'em in your pocket
Save 'em for a time when you're really gonna need 'em,
oh
The sharp knife of a short life, well
I've had just enough time
So put on your best, boys, and I'll wear my pearls.

Tears blurred my vision as I listened to the words.

I thought to myself, "Will that be me?" My chest felt

like it was caving in. I was terrified. I was literally

scared to death. Was this my legacy? I didn't want my husband to see me crying in my rearview mirror so I sunk down into my seat and gently wiped the tears away.

As I slipped out of the car door, I used the back of my hand to smear the remainder of wetness that remained. My husband inspected my face inquisitively with concern, as he held tightly onto our son. We walked into the house together, arm in arm.

I remained in shock for much of the day. I procrastinated in calling my Mom at eight pm. She wanted to hear how my doctor's appointment went, but she had her own issues to contend with. She was laid off from Foxwood's Resort & Casino after sixteen years of faithful servitude to the VP of Administration. At the same time she was diagnosed with a lung disease called Sarcoidosis.

My younger brother was just about to leave prison on a suspended sentence due to overcrowding and good behavior after doing his time. My sister was suffering from the endless cycle of infections from AIDS, fighting the disease for over twenty-five years, as a long term survivor. Like I said, ancestry like piss and vinegar! Pure strength.

The timing couldn't be worse. We had the house up for sale to move back to Connecticut. We had lived in Maine for eight years. And although we really liked it, I thought I could go back home and take care of my family, David would be closer to his family in New Jersey and I could go to Nursing School – which wasn't available nearby.

After all, I was the middle child. I was the good child. The Catholic student who never missed mass and whom the nuns praised as hearing the calling to being a nun, herself. I was the strong who always held it in and together. This vulnerable role was alien to me. Now I was the one who needed support. I was the one who needed to be taken care of. I felt weak and out of control.

I matter-of-factly told my Mom about my appointment. I think she was in shock, too. I tried to down play it, but I didn't do a good job. She started to sob. It made me feel sick inside that I was hurting my mother. She had no business even considering burying two of her children. It took her a while to get a hold of herself, but I tried my best not to cry. I think I ended up feeling like I was consoling my Mom, instead of vice versa.

It was the longest week-end of my life. It was Friday and I had to wait until Monday to find out any information as far as a neurosurgeon and the thought of possible cancer. My husband jumped onto the computer and looked up every neurosurgeon at Maine Medical Center in Portland, Maine.

There were a few posts on the computer and we looked up each doctor's credentials. My husband pointed to the computer screen and said, "I hope it's not this guy." I took a closer look. He looked like a crazy genius. I said, "That's probably the one we want. I want someone smart!"

While I laid in bed, I tried to think of any side effect of my brain that I had noticed. The only thing I thought of was that every once in a while I would hit a doorway with my left shoulder while at work. If I really thought about it, sometimes if I was cleaning off a stretcher at work or getting up from a chair, I would sometimes shuffle to the left.

It didn't happen often enough for me to call the doctor; just often enough to take notice. I thought it was old age. Or getting to an older age – ha. I was forty-two with three children and thought maybe that's when my coordination would start to be a little off.

I already spoke a little about Joseph, who was just a one year old. But I also had a son, Brett, who was serving in the Army in Afghanistan as a mechanic. He was a tall glass of water – and lanky. He tanned and freckled at the same time. Sometimes his hair was golden blond and sometimes golden brown. We butt heads, he and I. I was always in the need for control. He was always doing something reckless. I liked things neat. He liked things spread all over the floor.

But, boy, do I love him. I laugh now because our little arguments really don't matter. Not since I've stared death in the face. I have seen what is important. We may both be stubborn, but I pray for him every night.

Chapter 5

Monday, Monday....So Good to Me

I strummed the table with my fingers and waited for the phone call from the neurosurgeon. I still didn't know who it would be because it was a group. Around 11:00am was my time to call them if they hadn't called me. I waited until 11:05am in the hopes they would call me. I didn't know what information was passed along and I really didn't know what to say. My stomach was in knots. I just wanted someone else to handle this.

At 11:10am, I finally called. A woman answered and seemed confused about an appointment on Friday for me. I sighed. I knew this would happen. She asked me to spell my last name – twice. She said for some reason she couldn't find me in her computer system and would transfer me to someone else.

After a few moments, my call was transferred to a voice mail. It was the same office but another woman who eloquently spoke stating she worked for Dr. Florman, Neurosurgeon (I quickly scribbled his name onto a yellow sticky note) who was not available to take my call but to speak clearly and leave my name, number and the neurologist's name. She gave me a little more confidence that she knew what she was doing.

Literally five minutes went by and a frantic Vickie called me back. She was very apologetic about my first call and spelled out Dr. Florman's name and how to get to the Scarborough Maine Office. We made an appointment for 1/31/13. "Yes," I texted my husband, "it's the crazy genius!"

The neurosurgeon's office called me on Tuesday and said Dr. Florman wanted a CT-Scan image of my body before coming to our appointment. My husband flew into a panic. "Why does he want that?" He asked with trepidation.

"David, he's only doing his job. He needs to look and see if it spread, is all. Don't worry about it. I'm not worried about it." I mean, why would I have cancer riddled in my body? That's ridiculous, I thought to myself. I am way too young and healthy! This is probably an anomaly. I just got a 92% score on my health quotient from Maine Health. In response to health questions and in comparison to other women my age, I scored 92% better.

I called the neurologist's office and asked the lollipop guild (the secretary) if an appointment had been made yet for my CT-Scan. She was as aloof as her boss and blew me off saying she would call back. She never called back.

I called the next day and the same secretary said, "This isn't an easy thing. And she's dictating right now. I can't disturb her." I counted in my mind the number of times I interrupted a doctor who was dictating and swore I could have been rich had I selected another occupation. Again, I waited. Then I grew angry; this was my life we were talking about.

I couldn't see the neurosurgeon until I had my CT-Scan done. Finally, after I called the office for the third time, on the third day, it was scheduled. I evaluated the entire situation and decided to move my records to another neurologist in the same group; someone who was compassionate and cared about my life as much as I did.

That night, Dr. Stein of Neurology called me just to find out how I was doing at seven pm. I knew in an instant, that I had found the compassionate and wise physician that I was looking for. I had made the right decision. And along with the new neurologist, was the new secretary, Kathy, who was helpful and wonderful.

That night my daughter, Brittany, took me to the movies. I almost forgot about the brain tumor in the midst of watching one of the scariest movies ever! My biggest fear was screaming out in the quiet movie theater! She is the only girl I know who complains our house is haunted but insists on watching the scariest movies before bedtime.

The next day, I styled my hair with the proper 'pouf' and wore my best and most comfortable outfit. It was strange to hang out and wait as a patient in the emergency room. I kept wanting to do everything myself and felt guilty if I didn't handle the situation myself. I wandered aimlessly around the hallways and rooms saying hello to people I knew.

The nurses and doctors asked why I was in the emergency department holding a gallon of contrast. It was a moment. I paused and had to decide if I would share my news or keep it on the QT. I decided at that moment I would not carry the burden of a secret. If it was what my coworkers were suspicious of, I needed all the support I could get. I was blunt. "I may have a brain tumor; that's why I'm here."

People were shocked and supportive at the same time. I think there were many reasons that made it personal. We worked together as a family, for one. We were surrounded by disease like cancer and it didn't seem to touch us. However, about a two years before I started as a technician in the emergency department, another technician had a full blown seizure, an MRI and died six weeks later of a brain tumor. I literally sat in the same chair that she did.

Two years later our phenomenal colleague Dr. Tracy JalBuena was diagnosed with a rare case of Amyloidosis shortly after her father was diagnosed. I remember giving a sandwich to a good friend, Doug Barnette - an RN with a great sense of humor and cancer – who didn't eat that sandwich and died shortly after being treated at Maine Medical Center. We also received the frightening news that our young friend and EMT was diagnosed with cancer, as well.

With not much more to say, I hung out with my friends in the emergency department. My friend Jasmine kept crying. I tried to make the mood light while stroking her braid and said, "Don't cry for me,

Argentina." I felt totally fine! There was no reason for anyone else to be so upset. It hurt my heart.

The CT-Scan machine is a huge device that funnels you on a metal bed into and out of an x-ray machine. Depending on the test, you can either go head first or feet first; mine was feet first with arms above my head. Finally, after I drank my contrast over a two hour period and was ready to lie down and have my CT-Scan.

One of the x-ray technicians, Kary said, "Don't worry....you'll be fine." He went behind closed doors as my friend Jeff shot an IV into my arm. Jeff seemed fine and made small talk, but Kary seemed quiet, I sensed. I knew they were looking at my images in real time, as I had done so many times when I worked in the emergency room. After a few moments, my tests were done. Their lips were sealed.

I went back to the emergency room where Dr. 'Bob' Jorden and Dr. Tracy JalBuena said they could read the images with me. Instead, after ten minutes, Bob said he would meet with Dr. Charles Crans, my Guardian Angel on Earth, and review my case. How apropos - the two men who started with my case because of a herniated disc – were ending it, too.

Bob asked for a few minutes, then led me between the same radiology technicians who performed my test. The radiology technicians parted like the red sea and I felt a sense of foreboding.

I wrapped my arms around the radiologist, Dr. Charles Crans, and thanked him from the bottom of my heart for saving my life by identifying the brain lesion for more testing. He said, "You never want to see what I saw on your brain scan; especially someone of your age."

He paused and asked if I wanted to see the new CT-Scan images. I looked into the direction of the far corner of the room and saw a huge computer screen with the words, "Sherry Guarneri" and a split screen of a giant brain. It was my brain. The room was dimly lit. My heart was pounding. Did I want to see the results, I asked myself. Frankly, no; honestly, yes.

I took a seat next to Dr. Crans while Bob stood behind us. He asked if there was an image I would like to see first. I said I wanted to see my brain first, since no one had taken the time to review it with me so thoroughly. Slowly and methodically, Dr. Crans drilled through each image. He then opened the new CT-Scan. Gland by gland; muscle by muscle; bone by bone he interpreted each image. And then there it was.

So pretty. So white and shiny. A lung mass. A tumor. A lesion. So many words to call it; other than pretty. It sat by itself like a star in the universe of my right upper lung. We all sucked in our breath and stared at the screen in silence. "And there," said Dr. Crans, as he sat back in his chair for emphasis, "is your problem." Lung cancer. I mean, we didn't know until it was biopsied; but…lung cancer.

I immediately hung my head and thought, "I wish I was dead." All I could think of was that I would rather be dead than sick with my hands wrapped around a porcelain giant gagging for air. I would rather be dead than to tell the people that I loved I was going to die. I would rather be dead than to tell the people that were my friends that I had something as (what I thought of as) shameful as lung cancer.

Dr. Crans continued, "Your lungs are so healthy. I can tell you don't smoke." I quietly whispered, "I did smoke. I quit five years ago."

It was one of my proudest moments to quit smoking five years ago with the help of Chantix, a prescription through Pfizer. I was their spokesperson over four years ago. Pfizer marketing flew my husband and I out to Times Square, New York in December for me (and others) to speak with twelve reporters. I was told they may or may not run with the story. However, it was important for me to share it – even if I could change just one life.

I was met by magazine writers from Better Homes & Gardens to local newspapers. Some of the reporters took me aside and told me how proud they were of my accomplishments. Pfizer marketing paid for everything including air tickets, the Westin Hotel at Times Square and dinner, among many incidentals.

The following day, I gave interviews to several Human Resources officials, on behalf of Pfizer, to consider paying for Chantix for their employees. It was fun and exciting – especially our own time when we could window shop the most dazzling stores, see stars we normally saw on television and became entranced by the glistening and beautiful infamous Times Square Christmas Tree and the adjoining ice skating rink.

We even talked it up with a homeless guy trying to make a quick buck. I wanted to put him in my pocket and take him home. It was sensational. I thought our trip would go somewhere…it went nowhere. I had just wanted to help one person. Maybe I did. Not enough. Not me.

Dr. Crans continued, "Well, you can't tell. Your lungs are in excellent shape." My breathing was so shallow I couldn't hear it anymore. Always five steps ahead, I thought, how did it spread? That's all I could think of. I seemed to hold my breath every time his finger clicked the mouse.

He continued that the Adrenals looked good. The bones looked good. The lymph nodes looked good. That's good, right? Mom always told me that no one lives if it spreads to the lymph nodes (I didn't know much about cancer at the time).

The only thing left was the blood. And that, we wouldn't see. One of the million things I learned about cancer that I wished I hadn't was that a CT-Scan, MRI and PET Scan can only pick up cancer that is larger than the top joint of a finger.

Dr. Crans and Bob both told me I could beat this. They both said I needed a team of oncologists, radiologists and surgeons. Dr. Crans said something about getting a notebook and writing everything down. Me? I needed these people and these notebooks? I was still shocked. Was there hope? I doubted it. They're placating me, I thought. They know I'm dead.

Lung to brain…lung to brain…lung to brain. I was shocked. Bob walked me to the employee break room and hugged me. He looked stunned. Lung to brain…lung to brain…lung to brain…I walked to the car alone. I was so angry inside that I almost keyed a car right next to me. Well, I thought about it anyway. It was parked so close, I had to go in sideways into my car. But then I remembered something more important…lung to brain…lung to brain…lung to brain.

"David, where are you?" My voice cracked. "On my way home." He said. "I just got the results. I'll tell you when I get home. I love you." He said he loved me, too. I don't even think I cried on the way home. I was too shocked.

When I came inside the house, David was flying down the stairs, holding the baby. "Let's go upstairs." I said. I briefly saw that my daughter Brittany was sleeping on the air mattress in the living room. He was still holding the baby and we were huddled in our bedroom when we both started crying. God, I haven't even told him yet! "I need you to be strong, David. Please be strong. Please, Please."

"What is it? What is it?" He cried. He was almost on the floor. I grabbed him by the shoulder. "It's lung cancer! It spread from my lung to my brain!" We both started crying harder. He gave me the baby and went to the bathroom to get tissues and wailed and pounded on the sink.

My daughter came up, rubbing the sand out of her sleepy eyes and said, "Is that about you?" And pointed to the bathroom. "Yes," I cried. "Is it bad?"

She asked. I nodded, yes. She wrapped her arms around me and hugged me. Then David came out and we all hugged each other and cried out loud, in silence.

Later on, I asked David to call my mother and tell her the doctor's thought I had lung cancer. She was devastated and began to cry. I was listening upstairs with the bedroom door open and heard David say, "I can't live my life without her." I choked up the tears and quietly closed my door and laid in bed.

Hours had drifted by and David and I were lying in bed, looking at each other. I said, "I'm sorry." He said, "For what?" I said, "For picking me." David started to cry and said not to ever say that again.

The worst day of my life.

Chapter 6

Where oh Where is Scarborough, Maine?

The day I found out that I had cancer was my last day at work. After my vacation was paid, I was immediately put on short term disability and told it would transition into long term disability. The good news is that we would still have income coming in. The bad news was that I knew I would be on long term disability for a while and was told the cobra for health insurance would be almost twelve hundred dollars a month and my income would only be 60%.

We deliberately picked up secondary insurance for myself and the kids, in anticipation. Why didn't I listen to my grandfather and save my pennies for a rainy day?

I announced on Facebook to family and friends what I was going through and David and I started the websites 'Caring Bridge' for updates and 'Pay it Forward' which is a website that pays seven percent of the proceeds to other people who need financial security.

We drove over two hours to get to Scarborough – a long trip for two frazzled parents and one unhappy baby. Our daughter, Brittany, was in her junior year of high school and our son, Brett, was in the Army in Germany – soon to be leaving for Afghanistan. It's funny how children can all live under the same roof, but behave totally differently.

Brett never said a word. But he stayed with me overnight before being deployed to Afghanistan and I was able to kiss and hug him. Brittany didn't really want to talk about it, either. I think they wanted life to be normal. Normal routines; normal schedules.

We tried our best to keep Joseph occupied after we finally got to the office. We waited an hour and a half for the neurosurgeon to show up for our appointment. I wasn't so sure this was the best decision but I heard nothing but wonderful things about this doctor – including winning the Most Compassionate Doctor Award…compassion that I really needed about now.

After meeting with the medical assistant and the RN who asked me to perform neurological tests, Dr. Florman finally flew in. He was at least 6'7", with hair like Bob Dylan, wearing scrubs (maybe just coming from surgery) and moved and spoke like he drank six Red Bulls. I loved him immediately.

He quickly shook our hands and used the stretcher to plunk down three images from a computer. One was my brain. I immediately zeroed in on the bump that's on my nose and chuckled. He immediately zeroed in on the 1.0" (roughly) in diameter lesion at the back of my Cerebellem.

The second image was from a CT-Scan from PenBay Hospital that showed a bright star in the right upper lobe of the lung…suspicion of lung cancer. The third image was from an MRI which showed a bright star in the middle of the right lobe of the lung...another view for the suspicion of lung cancer. We simply wouldn't know if the lesion was cancer until it was biopsied on 2/11/13.

"Here's the deal." He pointed to the brain lesion on the first image. "That needs to come out." He pointed to the second and third image. "That lesion is coming out, too. But I'm a brain doctor, so someone else will be doing that."

"Now. If you're going to get a tumor in your brain, you've picked the right spot to get it in. The Cerebellum is about coordination. It does not make mental decisions. You will not have seizures because of it. But eventually you would have come to my office due to balance issues."

The questions shot out of my mouth like a .22. "How long will I be in the hospital? How long will I be in surgery? Do you have a team? What are the odds of it growing back? Will the Cerebellum close up? Will I have a plate and staples? What will I be like after surgery?"

He shook his head thoughtfully and answered each question. "You will be in the hospital for about three to four days. You will be in surgery for about two hours. Yes, I have a team. The odds of it growing back are small. The Cerebellum will close up around the hole over time. You will have a titanium plate and screws and dissolvable staples."

He continued, "After surgery it will feel like you're having somewhat of a stroke for a few weeks. You may need physical therapy. Since the Cerebellum controls muscle tone and coordination, balance and equilibrium, your balance and coordination will be affected. For instance, if you try to reach for a cup, your hand may move right by it. You may not be able to walk in a straight line. The biggest risk is that it grows back again."

Then David had his line of questions starting with, "How many times have you performed this surgery?" He always made me chuckle. I looked behind David holding the baby and I swear I saw the illusion of a man behind him…arms crossed….listening intently to the doctor.

I think it was my father, Kenny, who died in an auto accident at the young age of thirty-four. The rest of the time, I felt the presence of spirits alive and dead. It made me feel like I wasn't going to go through this alone.

After I was satisfied that Dr. Florman answered my questions (and David's), he suggested that we schedule a date in the calendar for surgery. I pulled out my handy-dandy calendar in which I was ironically the calendar girl for January for healthy living for Maine Health and showed him. He put his arms around me to hug me and said he would hang my calendar on his bulletin board over his desk to remember me. My husband said the doctor had tears in his eyes.

I did a quick neurological exam for Dr. Florman, once again feeling ridiculous but passed. The surgery was scheduled for the next Friday at Maine Medical Center on 2/8/13.

David shook Dr. Florman's hand and said, "Thank you. Thank you so much." I echoed, "Yes, you saved my life." Dr. Florman said nonchalantly, "It's what we do." David and I chuckled at the endearing but preposterous comment he made. If only David and I were brain surgeons!

However, I still had one more test that needed to be performed. A PET scan on 2/6/13, prior to my surgery, to look for more cancer. I remember feeling defeated. Couldn't people just leave my body alone for a while? I was afraid to have this test done. Brittany assured me it was okay by rolling her eyes.

She read that a PET scan stands for a positron emission tomography. It documents how the tissues and organs are functioning with the disturbance of cancer. A brighter spot picking up on glucose is usually an indicator of higher levels of chemical activity or cancer.

She continued that the test takes about an hour and a half to complete. The first part is sitting still for about a half hour. The second part of the test is to lie on a contraption similar to an MRI – however, there is no backing to the PET Scan – it's more like a CT-Scan.

Brittany was my little researcher. I honestly didn't want to know anything, at first. It was Brittany who would scan the information then give me the positive version. I would tell David her version and that's how we communicated. We were all afraid.

We drove to Scarborough a couple of days later to have the PET scan. It's available at my hospital but only every three weeks and the trailer was just there recently. My neurologist, Dr. Stein, said that wouldn't be quick enough and called Scarborough to have me do the testing there.

My PCP (Primary Care Provider) Dr. Kevin Davey had me come to his office and pick up Ativan to calm my nerves before testing. The only experience I had with Ativan was giving it to the poor souls who couldn't control themselves in the emergency room (another fallacy). Ativan can help with nausea, anxiety and sleep.

I took an Ativan one hour prior to the test and it worked just fine! I don't remember much of the test because I fell asleep, but in my experience the MRI was worse than the PET Scan because of Claustrophobia. It was now time to prepare for surgery and do something for myself before someone else got a hold of my body – like the body snatchers!

My friend Tracy told me about a great hairdressing place in Camden called The Cutting Edge. They do Chemo-cuts for free. It was time to start cutting. I met with my hairdresser, Sarah, as my husband and son looked on. Sarah was gentle, kind and sweet. She gave me the confidence to face cancer and I hugged her through tears when we left.

Cutting my hair made the cancer real. I couldn't face cutting it all off at once because I had long hair, so I had it cut short at first. I figured I could have Sarah layer it shorter a couple of times, then have my husband shave it when my hair started falling off.

People were coming forward and proving to be so giving and loving. It overwhelmed us. I still feel

uncomfortable when people want to help us. I
remember feeling guilty when people looked so sad,
looking at me. Did they fantasize that one day I would
be looking into the mirror of no return? Would I one
day no longer have a reflection? Would my children no
longer have a mother? I didn't know.

David told me about a tattoo he was interested
in getting. It was from the bible scripture of Jeremiah
30:17 and said, "For I will restore health unto thee, and
I will heal thee of thy wounds, saith the Lord." I
remember thinking, "Why? Who has cancer?" It never
occurred to me – at least for the first few seconds – that
it was me…I had cancer.

Chapter 7

Ready for Brain Surgery

Due to the pending snowstorm, we decided to leave a day early to get to Maine Medical Center in time for cranial surgery in the morning. I was the third candidate of the day and I hoped the surgeon's hands would be nice and warmed up when I arrived for brain surgery in the early afternoon.

All night and the next morning I listened to uplifting music on my I-Pod. Every time I looked out the window, I was reminded about my pending surgery as I looked through the snow and towards the lit sign across the street reading, Maine Medical Center. A part of me wanted this over with but I also worried the neurosurgeon would cancel my operation due to the weather.

The snowstorm was bad enough that there had been a nineteen car pile-up that we probably would have gotten caught up in on the highway that we luckily missed. We were disappointed that only two friends came for surgery; but so grateful to have the support of our good friends Sarah and Jasmine for moral support and prayer.

I received updates through-out the day from Dr. Florman's secretary that he was still in surgery. Around three pm, his secretary asked if I wanted to reschedule, per Dr. Florman who was still in his second surgery as it had more complications than expected. I panicked and asked her to tell him that we booked a hotel room and were right across the street. She called back and said to be ready for surgery around five pm.

At 5:30pm, I was whisked into a pre-surgery area and asked to undress and go to the bathroom (they didn't want to catheterize me, thank God, hoping my bladder would hold out). When I came out, David handed me a letter from one of my co-workers who was working on an ambulance that day. I read the letter from Craig. The tears welled up and reality set in when he described me like 'Radar' from the Army show MASH.

The Operating Room Nurse asked if I had an Advanced Directive to write my last wishes and to designate David as my medical power of attorney. My friend Sarah had the papers drawn up prior to surgery in case anything happened. There's a piece of paper you don't want to think about! But seriously, I was relieved it was done. I was asked about that piece of paper multiple times. I felt prepared in case anything happened. I also asked to see a Catholic priest during my recovery.

I was feeling nervous excitement at getting this thing out of my head. I know that sounds strange, but a voice inside my mind kept insisting, "Get it out!" It turns out the brain tumor could be more invasive than the lung tumor, so I was right in getting that out first. Call it shock, but I was silly with anticipation and fear but didn't shed a tear.

After a while, David and Brittany and my friends were all in the room with me before surgery. It really helped to make the time go faster. The Anesthesiologist, Dr. Abess, came in and I was elated to see that he also worked at the same hospital that I did almost two hours away! He recognized me immediately and said he was shocked to see the lesions. He immediately put my mind at ease.

Before surgery, Dr. Florman and the Anesthesiologist came in to describe the surgery. I asked

Dr. Florman, "Have you eaten today? I want a surgeon who is prepared and awake!" He laughed and told me a list of all the foods he ate, including a chocolate brownie.

I met the second Anesthesiologist who explained that I would be intubated for the procedure and placed on my belly. I had never been intubated and it scared me; I wished I hadn't known. Dr. Florman said my PET scan was sent to my oncologist, but he didn't see anything obvious. As quickly as he came, he left to get ready for surgery.

As we said our good-byes between family and friends, my eyes finally filled with tears and I hugged and kissed everyone in the room before I left. The Anesthesiologist pumped my veins full of fast acting drugs before wheeling me into a sterile room with several colleagues dressed in blue scrubs and a smile.

The second Anesthesiologist was behind me and Dr. Abess was in front of me. The second Anesthesiologist put an oxygen mask on my face. I said, "Are you putting me to sleep?" He smiled and said, "No." I remember we were talking about Cancun. I said I went to Cancun with my husband and it was great. Then I said, "God bless you. I said a prayer for everyone in this room." That's the last thing that I remember.

When I awoke, it was a few hours later. David had come in to check on me but I didn't remember. I just recall the embarrassment of the technicians (like me) trying to get me onto the commode. I was very wobbly and I had to hold the front of my head to feel support. After a minute, I told the technician I was going to be sick. She got me back into bed and I fell asleep.

Surprisingly, I was positioned on my back and my hair was still intact. Dr. Florman is the only doctor that does not shave hair off the head (he warned me not to color it either!). I recall one of the RN's looking at the stitches on the back of my head and saying with chagrin, "Oh, this has got to be Dr. Florman's handiwork; he never shaves head hair for surgery."

The hospital was packed with people so I ended up staying overnight in the recovery area until the technicians could find me a more private room the next evening. Unfortunately, in my new room, I had a roommate with dementia and a broken hip. Half the night I stopped myself from going to her bed, answering her call bell and finally answering her cries for help. It was exhausting. Every time I went to the bathroom, I needed assistance and a hand on my forehead. The RN's actually put a bed alarm on me. But otherwise I was feeling fine.

I am vaguely aware of a Catholic Priest doing the anointment of the sick after my surgery, as requested. I remember it was the only time the dementia lady clammed up and listened. The priest looked at the paper copy of my brain and the tumor that I had hung on the bulletin board as a reminder. He was incredulous. He stood by my brain tumor image for a while.

Dr. Florman described the surgery, though I was only half aware of reality due to surgery and drugs. He said he drilled a hole in my skull – almost centered in the back of it – then took out the brain lesion and all surrounding areas to ensure cancer cells did not exist. He did not see any other cancer in proximity. To close the incision, he used titanium pins and plates (I was officially bionic!). The surgery took place on 2/8/13; the lesion was to be biopsied on the day of discharge, 2/11/13.

I received word that the brain lesion was indeed cancer. It was Adenocarcinoma. It was probably the same cancer that was festering in my lung.

Adenocarcinoma is a non-small cell cancer. Eighty percent of lung cancers are non-small cell cancers, and of these, about 50% are Adenocarcinomas. Adenocarcinoma of the lung begins in the outer parts of the lung, and it can be present for a long time before it is diagnosed. It usually does not spread; though it did in my case. It is not hereditary to children. It is the type of cancer most commonly seen in women, usually under the age of forty-five and is often seen in non-smokers. Lucky me.

I stayed in the hospital for three days, which was long enough for me. I just wanted to go home. The doctor thought I should stay one more day but I even got up and showed him I could walk and go to the bathroom on my own. The only thing I had to do was hold pressure on my forehead when I got up from a downward position. Due to the fact that I had others in the house to help, he reluctantly allowed me to leave.

We stopped at the hotel to pay and were shocked and grateful to learn that our friend Julie P. had paid for the hotel accommodations. It was one less worry, especially since we were mostly depending on David's income to pay the bills. My income was 60% and less the shift differential. We pinched every penny. Thank God there were pennies from heaven because every time something catastrophic happened, someone would send us a check or cash in the mail or in person.

When I came home David had semi-permanently set up the air mattress for me in the living room so I could feel like part of the family. I slept downstairs, too, with David and Joseph so I didn't have to use the stairs. I was told the best way to recover the brain was sleep; and sleep is what I did!

Chapter 8

Stage IV with Mets

The date was 2/13/13, four days after cranial surgery and I was scheduled to meet with my Maine oncologist, Dr. Nadia Ramdin. After I found out about the tumors, I contacted my insurance company and asked if they would pay for a second opinion at Brigham and Women's Hospital/Dana Farber in Boston. They surprisingly said 'yes' and I was allowed over a hundred visits. My husband and I were scheduled to meet with Dr. David Jackman (Oncologist at Dana Farber) on 3/1/13.

I waited anxiously in the room with my husband, baby and our friend, Tracy from the emergency room. Dr. Ramdin was very abrupt about my report findings.

She said that she felt lung surgery was not an option because by reading the PET scan, it appeared that the cancer had spread beyond the lung and was hiding behind the chest plate.

If that were the case, and with aggressive therapy, I was considered to live for five years with Metastatic Stage IV lung cancer (due to the spread to my brain and possibly other areas). I was devastated. This was not anything that I had imagined. I thought that the cancer would take ten years off of my life. I cried and couldn't speak. They were the kind of tears that literally pushed out of my eyes and didn't touch my face. Hopeless tears. My friend found me some tissues.

I looked at my baby boy on my husband's lap and immediately thought I wouldn't be there for kindergarten or his first dance or the prom or his graduation. I thought about my other kids – older, but still needing their mother to walk them down the aisle. I thought about widowing my husband at forty-five. It wasn't fair. Life wasn't fair. It was too much. I cried out more tears; then I sucked them all back in. I was Sherry again – cool and composed. I told the oncologist to continue.

Dr. Ramdin wanted to start me on two and a half weeks of full brain radiation at the Harold Alfond Cancer Center in Augusta, Maine – forty five minutes away. I wished Augusta were closer; but it was keeping me alive. We had another option of going to another town but it was being remodeled and would push out chemotherapy two weeks. I would drive the forty five minutes. Who was I to complain?

I had time to think about doing radiation and to heal as my appointment in Augusta at the Alfond Center was on 3/5/13. In the meantime, I mentally prepared for my meeting with Dana Farber in Boston on 3/1/13.

While I waited for my next appointment(s), I had time to do background checks on both the radiation therapy center and their doctors and on the Boston hospitals and doctors.

Again, I called my Mom to keep her informed. I told her they thought I had lung cancer and would have about five years to live, if treated aggressively. My Mom started to cry, then sobbed, then wailed and eventually dropped the phone. My stepfather came to the phone – hearing the commotion – and told me my Mom needed about ten minutes before she could talk to me again over the phone. My heart sunk.

The second worst day of my life.

Chapter 9

I'm a Radioactive....Radioactive

We had an appointment with Dr. Healey, Radiologist at the Augusta Alfond Center to discuss our plan of action in early February. I liked that he graduated from Yale University in Connecticut – where I was raised. I didn't like that only forty percent of cancer patients went to the center for radiation. I also didn't like that the center was sparkling new. I had the feeling it was like the movie, "The Devil's Advocate", in that things weren't always how they appeared. As you may be able to tell I was somewhat skeptical by this time and my life situation.

I recall David parking the car and seeing three people get out of a car. They walked into the center in front of us and the patient reeked from the cigarette she was smoking. I recall feeling anger that I had to follow her in my condition; and compassion because I knew the power of addiction.

The secretary had no idea who we were and was obviously embarrassed. She asked us to have a seat and we waited patiently to meet with Dr. Healey. Finally, she led us to a sterile room where we waited to meet with the Radiation Doctor. I looked at my surroundings. The building had been built recently and it yielded a fresh smell and appearance.

We weren't waiting long when Dr. Healey came rushing in, after we met with the RN. He was another spitfire. I opened up my notebook, but didn't have time to write everything that was spewing out of his mouth. He gave me the three options for treatment but recommended the first one. He told me another thing I never knew about cancer and wished I hadn't. He said that chemotherapy does not go into the brain. The brain is its own structure. I immediately felt sick. I thought, if radiation didn't work…I was dead.

I said to him, "Will my hair fall out?" Just then, his office phone rung. Under my breath, I said, "It doesn't matter, I guess. I'm going to die anyway." He said quickly, "You are not going to die." Once he got off of the phone, he emphasized, "You are not going to die. What I want from you is, when one treatment doesn't work, you say, 'what's next?' and 'what's next?' I don't want you to give up. Can you do that for me?" I cried and said, "Yes."

At that point we rolled up our sleeves and decided to fight this thing. For some reason I felt safe and secure in his presence – like he would handle everything. I asked him to take it slow and let me write down our options, which he did.

One of the most important things we needed to do was to meet with Dr. Peveradi the following day at the Alfond Center to discuss my having a bronchoscopy / mediastinoscopy. It was imperative for my treatment to find out if the cancer had spread to behind my sternum; inquiring minds wanted to know – including Dana Farber.

We decided we would start full brain radiation treatments Monday – Friday, for two and a half weeks. Since it was Tuesday, Dr. Healey said the technicians would fit me for a radiation mask. I had no idea what that was, and didn't ask. I was completely overwhelmed with information.

Dr. Healey led us whistling to the common area. He told us to help ourselves to the refreshments. After pouring our coffee, Joe ran up to the fish aquarium and pointed to the orange and black spectacles. I sat down and took in my surroundings. The building was exactly what I had hoped for; it was fresh and new; yet I was still untrusting.

I had my first interaction with cancer patients in the waiting area. I was intrigued by the fact that some did not have hair and didn't seem to care. Others had horrible red rashes on their foreheads. Everyone was extra pleasant – humbled. I thought, "They are me; I am them." It was a prophetic moment.

"Sherry?" A smiling woman appeared. I said my good-byes to David and Joe. I was led into a dimly lit room. In the middle of the room was what looked like a CT-Scan Machine. I was asked to take off my jewelry and lie down. I said to be careful because I just had cranial surgery. It hurt to lie my head back.

Two technicians worked expertly to tattoo my face with ink for the next couple of weeks. One girl explained, "We're going to fit you with a mask. It'll kind of feel Claustrophobic." Oh, great, I thought. She continued that the mask would be wet because it needed to form to my face.

I tried to think of relaxing thoughts as the technicians left the room and scanned my brain through the wet mask. Inevitably, I imagined that my father was holding the hand on my left side, my mother-in-law was holding my hand on the right and Jesus was behind my head with His Majestic Hand at the back of my head, magnetically removing anything cancerous.

After about ten minutes, both technicians returned. But when they tried to take off the mask, it had stuck to my hair. They were exclaiming that they felt horrible but I told them it was okay because I was going to lose my hair, anyway. They pulled and pulled and one technician had to leave the room. Finally, the mask loosened itself from my hair and I was done. The technician said, "You're a tough cookie!" I smiled and said, "I've been told that."

By the time I left the building, I was already feeling more confident and hopeful. I was just a girl who needed a notebook, a pen and a plan.

Chapter 10

And I Called Him…Dr. Pavarotti

It was February, 2013. We met with Dr. Philip
Peverada in his Augusta office to discuss my having a
bronchoscopy and mediastinoscopy. The procedures
would require that I have my second surgery in the
Waterville Hospital.

The only way that David and I survived this
meeting was to keep telling ourselves that it didn't matter
what this surgeon said. That way it would give us our
control back – just in case he said it was bad news.

I sat down and immediately said to the surgeon,
"I don't want to know numbers. I don't want to know
how long I have to live. Please just tell me what I need
to do." I liked him immediately. His demeanor was
quiet and to the point. He was respectful of the fact I did

not want to know how much longer I had on this earth. He nodded his head and listened to me. He also advised me that he worked for many years at the same hospital that I worked in. It gave us a kinship.

He explained that a bronchoscopy is a procedure when a tube is inserted into the airway to look at the voice box, vocal cord, trachea and bronchi. Lung tissue can be biopsied through the bronchoscope for examination in the laboratory.

He continued that a mediastinoscopy would be performed at the same time. He said it was a surgical procedure to examine the inside of the upper chest between and in front of the lungs.

I asked how this procedure was done. He explained that I would be intubated, a small cut would be made in the neck just above the breastbone and a small scope would be inserted through the opening. A tissue sample (biopsy) would be collected through the mediastinoscopy and then examined under a microscope to see if the cancer had spread to behind my sternum.

Everyone was biting their nails over this test, so I figured it was pretty important and I scheduled the surgery. The question of the day: did the cancer spread from my lungs and up into my brain? Was the cancer in my lymph nodes? I would finally know with the results of this test. If it was positive, there was a question if Dana Farber would be interested in doing the surgery.

Before we left Dr. Peverada's office, he said, "I know you don't want to hear numbers but I just wanted to let you know that I have been doing Thoracic Surgery for many years and there are people who have lung cancer that has spread and they are doing quite well, living a full life. Also, it's favorable that the cancer did not spread through your lymph nodes. It's not the best news, but its better news."

A couple of days had gone by, and here I was again at the end of February for my second surgery in the Waterville Hospital. David told me he knew it would turn out okay because just before surgery he was behind a car and the vanity plate read, "Believe". He said I had to believe too. I changed into a hospital gown and sat on the bed. I met with the Anesthesiologists – both of which were women – and one of them took my hand and asked if I remembered why I was there. I said to see if the cancer spread. I'll never forget how she tenderly took my hand into her hand and crossed the fingers on her other hand and shook her head, 'no', while tears were in her eyes.

The last thing I remember is being rolled down the hallway in the stretcher and going into the operating room. The same number of people were there in their blue scrubs and smiles. Then I transferred from a comfortable bed to the cold, metal one and said, "I prayed for all of you." I remember smiles before waking up to my husband. I loved that Anesthesia was that painless!

The results were pretty quick. The cancer had not spread. It was not hiding behind my sternum. I think we all exhaled in relief. In conjunction with the license plate, "Believe", David saw another license plate after surgery, saying, "ItcnBdun" (it can be done). He had a premonition that the lung surgery would go well, too, because he saw the last vanity license plate, "SuzyQ".

Chapter 11

A Silver Lining

On March 1st, we drove the same day to Boston to meet with Dr. David Jackman. It's a three and a ½ hour drive from Maine to Boston and I had a lot to think about in that time. A change started to happen within me. I felt blessed to see the birds and the sky. I felt happy to just BE in the moment. I literally stopped to smell the roses. I was moonstruck over a bright green and red caterpillar scrunching across the tree bark. I love the smells, the sounds, the sun and the wind.

David didn't quite understand it all yet. All he saw was traffic. He was terrified the doctors would say I was a hopeless cause. I heard him grumble on more than one occasion about the other drivers.

I was thoughtful of what he said. Then I asked him, "David? What if suddenly the car in front of us slammed on his brakes? And you died. Would it matter that my cancer spread?" He said, "No." I continued, "Then stop thinking of the 'what ifs'. You could die. I could die. We don't know how much time we have." I think he got it. His shoulders once rigid, were now slumped. He smiled at me.

We wanted to save some money so David booked a cheaper hotel that was near the hospital, but it wasn't enticing. There weren't any parking spots except for across the street, where we ended up paying sixteen dollars to make sure the parking gate didn't extort our car.

Once we got into the hotel, we were ignored for the first five minutes. Finally, we complained about the parking – which they did nothing about – so we just paid for the room. We just wanted to lie down on the bed, watch cable and order dinner in. I knew it would be bad when the bar was attached to the hotel. I knew it couldn't be good when we opened the door to check out our surroundings and found furniture from the sixties.

I learned how painful cancer can be – for one reason due to pain meds and not being able to go to the bathroom. Pain meds are great to take away some of the pain but not so great when it slows down the intestine. I took a seat in the bathroom and heard a drunk guy singing (the walls were like loose-leaf paper). I hit the sink and cried. My life shouldn't be like this. But it was. Yeah, that's embarrassing – but my new truth.

The food tasted like crap and in the middle of the night once the bar closed mid-morning, a clawed intruder started scraping the grate above my head. I woke up David and for the next few hours he balled up clothes and tossed it at the grate – making it noticeably silent for a minute. Let's take a moment to shudder! I couldn't wait to leave that place! The next morning we didn't bother to use the snooze button – we were out of there! So much for my Pollyanna approach!

The next morning we hailed a cab but we weren't impressed by the taxi driver who took the round-about route to scam us from a taxi fare because he knew we were tourists, but we were thoroughly impressed by the introduction of the building. We got out of the taxi and looked up to see a steep skyscraper, glass windows and a beautiful piano ensemble singing to us the moment we opened the door. I felt like I was in Oz. I think I actually smiled.

We sat anxiously until the very pleasant physician's assistant came in and asked me a bunch of questions. She also did a brief neurological exam and was quite extensive with obtaining my history. We didn't wait long for Dr. David Jackman. Upon his arrival, he was accompanied by the renowned Thoracic Surgeon, Dr. Scott Swanson. I was impressed from the first time they walked into the room and spoke.

Dr. Jackman wore a nice, blue suit and Dr. Scott Swanson was wearing scrubs and a physician's coat. They both exuded warm smiles and compassion. They said that if the cancer did not spread (they would review the report), then they believed they could do what's called a VATS procedure on my right lung.

Dr. Swanson explained that VATS stands for Video-Assisted Thoracic Surgery to perform a Lobectomy. It's a minimally invasive surgical technique used to diagnose and treat problems of lung cancer. During this surgery a tiny camera and surgical instruments are inserted in the chest through small incisions. The images are available via a video monitor to guide him through the procedure. In my case it was used to remove an entire upper lobe from my right upper chest cavity.

I clearly remember Dr. Swanson leaning up against the wall and listening intently to me saying I didn't think I would live anyway because it had spread to my brain…I may have even relinquished a tear or two. Dr. Swanson said very thoughtfully and emphatically, "You are not going to die. You will be fine. We are not looking to treat this; we are looking to cure it."

That gave me an inexplicable amount of hope. I remember the surgery was scheduled three weeks later, which we thought was pretty quick. Dr. Swanson assured me that he didn't believe the lung cancer would spread before surgery. I also recall I liked him because I kind of thought he looked like Leslie Nielson from Airplane and that movie meant a lot to me and my stepfather, "…and don't call me Shirley!"

Dr. Jackman advised me that he was now my primary oncologist. He appreciated that if there were any orders, they be passed through him. He would also design the chemotherapy order. We shook hands on our agreement and I left feeling like I was floating on air! All I wanted was hope. I got hope.

Chapter 12

Good-bye Multitasking

It was my first day doing full brain radiation for two and a half full weeks. Just prior to treatment I met with a Priest who blessed me praying for the anointment of the sick. It was the first time I had been in a church in some time. It's funny how jail and dying bring you closer to God. The priest had a great sense of humor. I needed positivity all around me.

During Radiation I wore loose clothing and removed all of my jewelry. If you know me, then you know that removing make-up and jewelry is a big thing for me! At first during treatment I made sure that everything matched, my make-up was flawless and my jewelry was worn until the technicians called me in.

What a difference from then until now. Now I just make sure I'm wearing the same color flip-flops!

The administration gave me authorization to enter through the back door for privacy. I was almost always escorted by my husband or an ER (emergency room) nurse. Every now and again I would hear the whistle of Dr. Healey and smile. He was so positive it was contagious. I watched Joseph watching the fish and remembered how fresh and new that was to me once. I started to have flashes of happier times at my grandparent's house like catching frogs from their pond and picking blueberries from the garden.

"Sherry?" A young woman asked, breaking my daydream. I smiled and told David and Joe I'd be back soon. I was rerouted to a room different from where my mask was placed on my face. The radiation machine was like an overgrown CT-Scan. Three women awaited my arrival and gently placed me on the metal bed that was covered by a blanket.

One of the ladies said, "Sherry, we'll be in the other room for about four minutes. You shouldn't notice a smell or anything, but some people are sensitive and do. We won't be long and will be watching you. If you have any problems, just raise your hand." I nodded.

And with that, she snapped the mask over my face. It made me feel a little like Hannibal Lector and I had no idea what to expect. I closed my eyes and could hear the machine turn on. I squinted and could barely make out a blue laser scanning my brain. I must be one of those sensitive people because I immediately smelled a mechanical smell. It stuck to the inside of my nose and I breathed it in on the way home. It made my stomach queasy.

I was especially grateful for the interruption of the constant flow of soft rock music playing overhead. Every lyric seemed to be written just for me. Again, my father was holding my hand on the left; my mother-in-law was holding my hand on the right and Jesus was behind my head with His Majestic Hand magnetically pulling out the cancer from my brain.

At least the therapy wasn't that long. After four minutes, the ladies came in and helped me off of the metal bed. In another forty five minutes, I was home. The trip wasn't long because I usually ended up sleeping most of the way.

The list of long term effects for full brain radiation is extensive. I was told by several doctors my cancer would be treated very aggressively due to my age and I retorted, "Bring it on." But I wasn't feeling so confident after each mode of therapy.

For instance, I had no idea that the effects of radiation therapy could begin days to months after completion. For me, the effects of full brain radiation was hair loss (in clumps and can be permanent), skin irritation on my hairline, hearing problems because the wax in my ear had become hardened (looking like white paper), memory issues (sometimes forgetting words), and brain swelling (due to a lack of dexamethasone).

As a matter of fact, I was lucky the first day of radiation treatment that I wasn't alone. I started to vomit and couldn't hold anything down. Someone handed me a wastepaper basket. I had a migraine-like headache. One of my friends called the doctor after hours and he immediately put me back on the prescription dexamethasone – which he had taken me off of because he said it could sometimes mask the growth of a tumor. However, in my circumstance, my brain began to swell.

My friend, Donna, rushed to the pharmacy and picked up the prescription while I didn't feel better until hours later when my friend, Sarah, coaxed dexamethasone down my throat using some bread and water. Not the first time my life had been saved.

I was now doing the medication dance for up to fourteen pills in a day. It was so confusing that David took over the task and gave me my medication daily. Medication wasn't his only task. Our roles were completely reversed and I was no longer was able to multi-task, remember things short term or walk in a straight line.

Once the control freak, I had to relinquish it to David who was now the caregiver for our children, the cleaner, the grocery shopper, the chef, the chauffeur, the caretaker for me and the bill payer. We used to argue once a year; now we bickered almost daily. But we loved each other so much that our anger didn't last long. I am truly lucky and grateful to have my husband and best friend support me through this.

I guess the biggest issue was eventually getting a ride to radiation and back since my husband had to go back to work after a couple of months. My four Angels – Donna, Sarah, Jasmine and Tracy – worked out a travel schedule for me. Every day a nurse from the emergency room volunteered their time to take me to and from radiation treatment. They also watched Joe because David and I hadn't had daycare in the past – we worked opposite schedules. Tracy set up the Meal Train for us so we didn't have to worry about making dinner.

My second biggest issue was remembering anything thanks to short term memory loss and relearning to walk (in hallways and not the walls so much). When I was tired, I had a habit of stumbling backwards and losing my words. But I was too stubborn to shower with my husband helping me or asking for help. Instead, I left the door unlocked and the shower curtain open – in case I fell.

My third biggest issue was running my hands through my hair and seeing a clump of it between my fingers. I decided to have Sarah from the Cutting Edge cut it again. The third haircut was a buzz cut – compliments of my husband. I didn't want straggly hair and I wanted to be in control of losing it.

I told my husband I was ready and he put a towel around my shoulders. I sat in a chair and watched myself in the bathroom mirror as he buzz cut the whole thing. I didn't cry. He promised me he would cut his, too. He didn't. We used humor a lot to get us through difficult times so when he ran his hand through his hair and said, "But it'll be so short." I sarcastically said, "Really?"

I would often sleep on the way to Radiation and back and most hours in between. I was grateful for my air mattress in the middle of the living room. I slept on that thing day and night. I called it my communal bed. I loved to sleep on it at night with my baby and husband or lie across it and gossip with my daughter. It was hard for me to eventually put it away.

One time during Radiation a woman approached us and asked what kind of cancer I had. I told her lung to brain. She couldn't believe it because the woman she had brought to Radiation had the same kind of cancer. While I was in Radiation the lady pressed something into David's hand and asked that he convey to me that I would be okay. She said she held onto a cross that said, "Faith Can Move Mountains." Every time after that, I put the token into my pocket and believed I could do anything through faith and repeated the phrase.

Finally, on the last day of Radiation, I met with Dr. Healey and my friend, Kelly. Dr. Healey showed me my brain images and said that he was thrilled to report that I was clear of brain tumors. Additionally, he said full Radiation Therapy had been completed and he would see me again when I was eighty years old!

Chapter 13

Good and Getting Better

On 3/7/13, I met with my oncologist, my husband
and our son, Joseph. I was disappointed that there was
only one outdated lung cancer specific book in the
library among dozens of breast cancer books. Yes; to
this day many people see the handkerchief on my head
and my youthful appearance and immediately lower their
eyes and assume I have breast cancer.

I told my husband I wanted to go to the gift shop
and buy him a white and silver bracelet for lung to brain
cancer and a pin for myself. I was disappointed again to
find only pink ribbons. Breast cancer is just as important
as any other cancer. As a matter of fact, I believe that
cancer is cancer. However, I made a promise to myself
that I would be a part of the change for people who

suffered from all cancer, especially lung cancer. There is no shame in cancer.

So when Chris Wytock and the Rockland Fire Department offered to sponsor a Spaghetti Dinner and Silent Auction for me, I was dumbfounded. Julie P. and Kelly helped to put it all together. All of my friends and family were planning on attending September 21, 2013.

I wanted to use this opportunity to set up a couple of tables. One table for homemade white/silver ribbons for lung and brain cancer and purple ribbons for cancer (which I made and, of course, forgot to bring! I decided to use the ribbons for Lung Cancer Awareness Month in November). We also planned on setting up another table for people to volunteer for the American Red Cross Blood Drive and Bone Marrow Treatment. I also planned to bring literature and brochures with me regarding lung cancer.

This time when we met with the oncologist, instead of the bad news from the last time that I had five years for the quality of life, I was given wonderful news – after reviewing the bronchoscopy, it was determined that surgery could be performed on my lung. The doctor told me to smile because it was good news, but I was guarded to feel excitement. After all, I never knew that I had cancer. It taught me to question my reality.

We were scheduled to meet with Dr. Swanson on 3/15/13, but the secretary contacted David and asked if we could come sooner. After he said yes, he panicked. He asked if I knew why they wanted to see me early. Was there something wrong? Did they see cancer lurking in the shadows? It's just one example how the little black cloud constantly follows our family.

Just then, the phone rang and it was Dr. Swanson's secretary again to say that it was not an emergency to move the appointment. The doctor wanted to know if I could come to the office earlier because he wanted to televise my impending surgery for educational purposes and needed me to sign off on paperwork.

David asked me and I agreed. We arranged to drive to Boston the day before our appointment to meet with my Thoracic Surgeon, Dr. Swanson. This hotel was better than the last, although I still heard voices at 2am between a security guard and a drunk patron. Hello, big city! Boston was going through a cold snap and the wind was blustery, almost carrying us away like Pooh Bear.

As we checked into the hotel, David was waiting at the front desk and I became aware of a well-dressed lady standing next to me with her credit card extended. I pulled down the handkerchief on my forehead and noticed her staring at me. I don't think she realized it, but she said out loud and under her breath while looking at me, "Oh my God."

At first I was really subconscious about my multi-colored handkerchiefs (compliments from my friend Tracy). I was truly scarier without wearing one! I looked like a bald eagle! I tried to always wear head scarves in public. One time a visiting nurse came without my knowledge and I practically screamed when she saw me through the window. People would stop and stare or their children would ask why I had a mask on. David would get really upset. But I told him that I thought people were looking at our baby and then me and felt compassion.

After a while, it became second nature. I felt proud to be bald. Instead of looking down, I held my head up proud and looked people in the eye like, "Yeah, that's right. I have cancer." When I dropped Joe off at daycare, the little kids finally stopped staring and asked me why I was wearing a head wrap. I finally took it off and asked if they could massage my head with their magic fingers to make my hair grow back.

I have never been the wig type of girl, although I was told they run about seven hundred dollars and our insurance paid for it. I much preferred at first to wear something over my head and later on to wear nothing over my head while in the house – until my husband started referring to me as Friar Tuck and Susan Powers, the motivational speaker, "You can do it!" – Very funny, David.

Excited about the next day, we decided to go to sleep early, pick up something to eat at the Prudential Building and window shop. We also saw the movie, "The Fighter" with Marc Walberg. It was a good movie to keep my mind off of things. However, I didn't sleep well that night.

The next morning we were star struck with Brigham and Women's of Boston which was even nicer than Dana Farber. We used their valet service and walked into a hospital that looked like the Westin Hotel. People were bustling, vendors sold coffee and we were completely lost for a short time until we found the X-Ray Department, as requested by Dr. Swanson.

The Radiology Room felt a little like a cattle-drive as they called one person after another. After my two images were done – always a chest x-ray of one to the front and one on the side, we waited for Dr. Swanson to see us in his office.

I sat on the examining table, David sat with Joe on his lap and Brittany was in school. It wasn't long before Dr. Swanson's assistant and her colleague entered the room. She asked me to catalog what had happened to me.

I told her about the day I found out that I had cancer, brain surgery, the bronchoscopy and the radiation. She put a gentle hand on my shoulder and said, "Do you know how strong you are? I cannot believe you just gave me all of your history. People who just had brain surgery are not able to do that." I smiled. Really, I thought to myself? I guess I was harder on myself that what I originally believed. She told us Dr. Swanson would be right in and left the room.

While I waited with renewed confidence, I cautiously opened up a lung cancer pamphlet. For the first few months I flat out refused to read about it because I was afraid it would determine my fate. My grandfather saw his regular doctor for a routine physical and was told he had cancer that had spread from the colon to the liver and he would die six months later – he died six months later. I refused to have this as my destiny.

However, I figured it was time to learn a little more about my disease. I started to read passages out loud to David and quietly to myself. I had purposely not reviewed the lung cancer literature because I knew it to be bad. However, I clung to the notion that at this point, I needed optimism. I needed hope.

One section read that, although not everyone is the same, lung cancer kills more people every year than any other cancer. Like an addict, I continued to read that lung cancer kills at an earlier rate – typically within five years (and this is as long as it hasn't metastasized). I started to cry. Five years; METS IV (is all I could think of over and over).

Just then, Dr. Swanson and his team came in. Perfect timing. Dr. Swanson asked how I was doing. With tears rolling down my cheeks I said I was okay until I read the pamphlet and saw my life expectancy. The room grew uncomfortably quiet. I made the decision that instead of keeping everything inside, I would take a chance and share my greatest concerns out loud. No more secrets.

The first question I had was if I would die in my sleep. Dr. Swanson made an inquisitive face, then said no. I asked if he thought the cancer had gotten bigger. He said in his experience, the lung tumor would probably not grow or not grow more than a millimeter or so. He said, "If it has gotten larger, I will call you on your cell phone." I was impressed by this because it was a Friday afternoon and meant he would be calling us after hours.

He swiveled around and looked at my x-ray images. He said they looked fine – just like the others prior. Then he thoughtfully turned around and said to Joseph, "Your Mommy is going to be fine." I felt a little embarrassed about bringing up my fears; but also relieved that he was able to answer my questions. I trusted him. People found it hard to believe that he was doing my surgery because he was the, "Top Guy".

I signed all the paperwork to give my authorization to air my surgery for a tutorial. Anytime I was asked to help and share in my grief, I did it. I wanted to spare the next person or help them through it. The lung cancer surgery was scheduled for March 25th.

I met with a technician who took some blood-work and performed an EKG. The Anesthesiologist came in and reviewed my documentation. He assured me the VATS Surgery should be about four hours. I would probably stay in the hospital for four days. Everything else looked great in my chart. I found that I just couldn't be happy or grateful or relieved. I kept waiting for the other shoe to fall.

Chapter 14

I Miss My Family

They say that the third time is a charm and it was with our hotel rooms! Our friend Donna was coming later that night. She (and anonymous others), had paid for the Hampton Inn Hotel and transportation (though they won't fess up to it). The hotel had a little snack shop, free meals, a shuttle, a pool and workout room and our own parking. Brittany stayed in the hotel room while my mom and stepfather were due to arrive on Tuesday or Wednesday. Surgery was scheduled for Monday. We had the week-end to unwind.

Monday morning came too early. This was a surgery I was not looking forward to, but I was still in good spirits. It felt good to have this imposter out of my chest. I worried my oxygen level would be low and I'd have to use oxygen at home. I worried the pain would be too great and I might panic if I couldn't breathe. But none of those things turned to fruition.

Truthfully, I don't remember much of the pre-surgery because I was under sedation but I believe I 'blessed' the surgery team again before they started. I just remember a brief moment when I was awe-inspired by the cleanliness of the machines and the number of blue gowns and their smiles before I was intubated.

About four hours later, Dr. Swanson let David know that everything turned out better than fine and they had high hopes for my speedy recovery.

My eyes blinked open and I realized where I was. I was in the right side of the room and the room-mate to another lady who was older and had the same surgery on the left lung. It wasn't her first time for the surgery. I cautiously put my hand over my right side to feel for bandages. I felt fine as long as I wasn't moving. Unfortunately, the best way to recover from lung surgery is movement. I had to start to get things moving by later that day. If I had a dime for every person who told me to walk, I'd be a rich lady!

It was the hardest surgery for me. Yes, even tougher than brain surgery! The pain was excruciating and I often pushed the button for the PCA (patient controlled analgesia) for Morphine. I had three very small incisions around my ribs and right arm, including a chest tube. It's hard to believe that anything fit in through there – let alone instruments and a tumor! The tumor was removed through one of the small incisions and into a bag for further genetic testing. I had staples in the wounds removed a few weeks later.

It was an excellent hospital, but the interruptions gave no rest to the weary. It seemed that they had a separate technician, doctor, hospitalist, housekeeper, RN and specialist scheduled to come in by the hour – if not more. There were so many people coming in that I didn't know who they were and often looked for a badge. One drugged thought I had was, "What if this person just came off the street and they're demented asking me questions?" Worse yet, "I'm answering them!"

I had several nurses that were extremely compassionate and smart. I just didn't like them too much when they made me sit up and cough while they hit my back to loosen up the phlegm to prevent pneumonia. It was so hard to find the energy to cough. And I noticed that my ribs seemed to rub against the inside of my lung cavity which was a little uncomfortable. I didn't know if that would be forever.

I suffered through intermittent chest pain, numbness in the top of my right arm and a somewhat constant cough. However, my oxygen saturation remained at 100% - that's like getting an A+ on a test.

A few times a day I had to get up, freshen up and go for a walk – dragging everything with me! I felt a little ridiculous carrying around IV poles and walking via a stand up wheelchair at .2 miles an hour! The first day I looked like typical Sherry – made up; handkerchief in place. The second day – no make-up. The third day – no handkerchief. The fourth day – no make-up, no handkerchief with black circles around my eyes. I started out strong, anyway.

Things started to go from bad to worse, in my philosophy. First of all, I was asked if a student nurse could help. At first I was more than happy to help someone have a teaching moment. However, I soon wished I could have taken it back, because it became too much.

After my x-ray (which came out great), the student and the nurse started playing around with my suction machine. Suddenly, I couldn't catch my breath.

I looked at David in a panic. He announced I couldn't breathe. I literally felt the remainder of my right lung collapse. It was so painful. The suction had been removed from my lung and it immediately deflated.

For the next few hours I was told the lung would need to come up on its' own. The pain of the cramps was indescribable as the lung crept up its' cavity. At one point, when I was alone, I hung over the bedrail and cried. Was this worth it, I asked myself. Tears escaped from my eyes and hit the floor.

It was also hard because my friend, Donna, and my family couldn't stay as long as they wanted to because of the baby. It made me feel alone and scared. I asked to speak with a Catholic Priest. He woke me up and spoke with me for a while then said another prayer for the anointing of the sick. I was hoping that God could get me through this. I kept mumbling the mantra of my friend, Tracy, "Healing is happening".

On Wednesday, I woke up to my mother and stepfather next to my bed, smiling at me. It was like eating chicken noodle soup! It was so good to see my family. My Mom, Linda, brought some scarves for my head and words of encouragement. My stepfather, Doug, kept repeating that all would be okay because he had friends upstairs (both his parents passed). My parents had the opportunity to meet with Dr. Swanson. I wish they could have stayed longer.

The next day I was in even more pain. I felt something like gristle at the bottom of my lung. I was circled by Dr. Swanson and several more people. They discussed what could be wrong. It wasn't long before the Physician's Assistant told me to suck in my breath and hum while she removed the suction from my chest.

She placed another chest tube in and stitched it into place, right as I lay in the hospital bed. This seemed to help the machine to suction better and it helped me initially from the pain of air getting into my chest cavity. The group hypothesized that there may have been a hole in the suction tube connecting to the chest tube.

After my x-ray the next day I was told we had another problem. It appeared that 30mls of fluid was sitting on top of my lung and looked like Pleurisy (inflammation of the tissue of the chest wall). I asked what could be done about this. I was told that another x-ray would be taken the next morning because sometimes the fluid dissolves into the body. Luckily, the next x-ray proved the lung was clear and ready to finally heal.

I had blood-work drawn every day. And almost every day I was low on electrolytes and minerals like potassium (Hypokalemia) and magnesium. The RN's had me drink something that tasted like pure salt mixed with cranberry juice. I also wore venodyne boots (leg boots) and had daily Heparin shots in my stomach to prevent blood clots.

Cancer is not pretty. I recall one time on the second day when the Physician's Assistant sat next to me in bed and asked how I was feeling. I had just eaten a Greek Salad and told her I wasn't feeling too...too...and with my hand over my mouth I started to wretch.

I could tell that she was either new or had never done this before but she ran out of the room to fetch a pink bucket for me to get sick in. She didn't make it; and neither did I. I got sick all over the blankets on my bed and it even flew up into the handkerchief on my head. I add this story for humor and to let people know the truth about cancer. It's not just about tee-shirts, races and ribbon lapels. It's real. And it's never pretty.

The following day I was told I could have the chest tube out. The Physician's Assistant and a technician came in. I never met the technician, but I held her hand like I was in a life raft, while the Physician's

Assistant told me to hum a tune again. She pulled out the chest tube and I felt immediate relief.

She said I was a very strong woman. She was a really nice person – I don't remember her name. But she was kind, smart and funny. I should also add that Dr. Swanson was an amazing surgeon. He visited me every day, if not a couple of times a day. I was so glad that God used his hands as instruments to heal me. I was also impressed with the entire Thoracic Surgery Team. They were genuinely concerned for me.

I was asked a few times if I would like to sign a Pneumonia form to give permission for the shot, before leaving. I was also asked to have the Flu Shot, but I actually had the flu right before I was diagnosed with cancer. Since Pneumonia was a specific complication of the surgery, I finally decided to have the shot. I was asked if a student could give the shot to me under the instructor's training. I said, okay. The student asked if

I was ready and I nodded. She counted, "1...2...3", and only put the needle in a quarter of the way. "I can't do it!" She cried.

I couldn't believe it. The instructor took over and gave me the shot. The student was very apologetic and I forgive her but I was in so much pain by that point. It was the kind of pain that just makes you shake from head to toe. I tried to make it a teaching moment and told her I went through the same thing too – being afraid to do Phlebotomy because I was afraid of hurting the person. Then I realized in the end I was helping the person. Her eyes began to tear and she thanked me. I knew she would make a good RN someday because she cared.

All was well except for the fact I could not urinate. I tried and tried and tried. I think I may have had stage fright because the bathroom was on my roommate's side. This did not go well with the hospital but I understand that Anesthesia can slow down the bowels and the kidneys. I was catheterized more than once.

Finally, on the fourth day when I left the hospital, I was told I could leave but not without a catheter to be removed three days later by my Primary Care Provider. I was so disappointed but couldn't wait to get out of the hospital and to the hotel and eventually home – I would have agreed to a root canal by that point! Not that the hospital wasn't great. I just wanted to go home.

The inevitable question was asked, "Could a student put in your catheter?" I reluctantly said, okay. Stupid, stupid, stupid! First of all, it was completely embarrassing; I felt like I was ninety years old using a catheter – no offense to ninety year olds! After all, I was an emergency room technician and helped to insert them a thousand times. Second of all, it was during my menses (sorry, guys), even more embarrassing. Third of all, she tried three times and couldn't do it. Then the instructor had to show her how it was done; and the instructor tried twice before getting the catheter to work.

I was wheeled down to my car with the catheter bag attached to my leg. I hated that thing! I was constantly worried I would pull on the tube and it would rip me apart from the insides. If I knew how to remove it, I would have. It's just one more stressor that I didn't need. That's the truth.

I wore the catheter over the week-end until I ended up with a terrible sore throat, the day we left Brigham's Hospital that wouldn't go away. I showed my friend Tracy my throat. She said she thought I should go to the emergency room. They not only removed my catheter (thank you, Tracy & Kelly) but I was found to have thrush and cold sores in the back of my mouth.

I was shocked. My sister, Lisa, had Thrush often because of AIDS. And cold sores I never knew I had – I thought for sure it was Strep Throat – I had white pustules all over the back of my throat. However, I was told that people with low immune systems can actually break out with Thrush and cold sores from their own system.

Thrush is a yeast infection in your mouth – for lack of a better term. I never thought in a million years that I would experience this. It can be found as a raised whitish color on the sides and back of the tongue. I've only had it once but I knew something was wrong because when I brushed my teeth and my tongue, my tongue hurt. If it goes on for too long, it can actually go down your throat. A free piece of physician's advice: if a tongue depressor cannot remove the white patch on the tongue, it's probably Thrush.

Cold sores can also look like Strep Throat. I had them covering the back of my throat. It hurt to eat and talk. After simple antibiotics, both infections were treated with Magic Mouthwash and lozenges. I learned that people with cancer often get Thrush and mouth sores and should swish and spit daily.

I should add that the second I got home from the emergency room I tried the bathroom. Yay! I was so excited to text the girls that my kidneys were working just fine! One of my cancer tee-shirts reads, "Fight like a Girl!" One of my girlfriend's texted back, "Pee like a Girl!" My friends could always make me laugh, even in the most difficult of times

Chapter 15

Surgery Number Four

On 4/21/13, I ended up going to the Emergency Department for a horrible stomach virus. Dr. Jorden (Bob) said he was ordering a brain scan and an x-ray. I was having headaches and chest pains. It brought up all kinds of not so old memories. The virus was so bad by this point that for days I had only been vomiting bright green bile.

I wrung my hands for an hour and found out that both tests came back clear. Huge sigh of relief. The emergency room gave me meds and I didn't get sick again from the virus. However, I was told to wear a mask to ensure I didn't pick up viruses since I was about to start Chemotherapy. This was really difficult with a one and a half year old; he seemed to pick up on every virus imaginable, as did I!

Joe loved daycare, which we called, 'school'. He learned to say more words and socialized more. It amazed me that he would take off on his own and actually look forward to going to school, learning and seeing his friends. The only downside was the illnesses.

The first few months Joseph was there, he was sick with viruses and double ear infections. He constantly had a cough and a runny nose (which meant David, Brittany and I got a cough and a runny nose). But, it was 'school'. He loved it. I adjusted to the mask. And when I got sick, I got sent home from Chemotherapy. The first time I cried. After that, it was just part of the process. I was sent home about three or four times – not bad for four months of Chemotherapy.

Mid-April we were scheduled to meet with Dr. Swanson to remove the stitches in my side. However, on April 15th, the Boston Bombing unfortunately happened. We watched CNN in horror and hoped the criminals would be caught. On Friday, April 19th, I contacted Brigham and Women's Hospital and asked if my appointment had been cancelled or not due to the bombing. One brother who allegedly did the bombing died on Thursday. The police were still looking for the other brother on Friday. The hospital advised me that we could still drive down for the appointment – after all, they were a hospital and hospitals don't close.

We were in Portland, Maine – about two hours away from home – when we received a call from Brigham and Women's – the hospital had been shut down. Actually, Boston had been shut down to look for the lone bomber who was still alive. We turned around to go home.

We hoped the bomber would be found, but I worried the stitches would stick and grow into my side. The first appointment we had was about two weeks after surgery and we weren't able to make it to Boston. If we couldn't make the third week after surgery because the hospital was closed, we were looking at four weeks with the stitches in my side.

However, we eventually met with Dr. Swanson and members of his team the following Friday after the bombing. The alleged bomber had been incarcerated and the streets were relatively safe. My husband and I drove along slow to see the wave of bouquets, pictures, people and letters regarding the people who died and the people who were injured in the bombing. God bless all of you, I thought. My problem seemed so insignificant. Then I was reminded that every soul has a journey.

Finally we met with Dr. Swanson and his team. The technician removed my stitches without much pain, in no time and the tiny scars looked healthy. A physician who worked with Dr. Swanson came in and we made idle chit-chat. I reviewed my entire cancer story with him and he seemed intrigued.

Just then, Dr. Swanson came into the room. It was so good to see him. He said the x-rays looked fine and I could start Chemotherapy. He said they may or may not order direct radiation after chemo, but he didn't think I would need it. He also said he thought he got it all and that I was cured, though he still wanted chemo because the cancer cells had traveled through my bloodstream. He asked that I return after chemo in four months to meet with him and Dr. Jackman.

As a signature good-bye, I gave him (and his staff) a delicious cake from a Maine bakery and said, "Thank-you" on the top of it. I also said, "Well, I am tired of hearing how renowned and wonderful you are…people can't believe you did my surgery…so, I am giving you my signed calendar so you'll remember that I am also a celebrity."

We laughed and he turned red. He looked at my Maine Health calendar picture and said he would hang it above his desk so he could always remember that smile. It made me smile, too, to be able to do something for someone else – and not to have the spotlight on me for a change.

On 5/3/13, I was supposed to start Chemotherapy. The doctor(s) ordered Cisplatin and Navelbine. This is a poisonous combination but if it worked, it meant the cancer would be strangled from multiplying itself and my healthy cells could eventually grow.

High dose Cisplatin had a lot of side effects. Almost every dose that I had resulted in nausea and vomiting about four days later. I lost a lot of weight –

twenty five pounds and counting – because the chemo changed my taste buds. Most times when I looked, or even smelled food that I loved - like chicken, chocolate and ice cream - I dry-heaved. I just couldn't eat. The only thing to compare it to is pregnancy.

I learned that the chemo drugs take some time to elevate in the bloodstream. I often tested abnormal for a low white blood cell counts – or fighter cells – which can give me the risk of infections. This meant wearing masks that made me sweat. It meant no germ infested areas like daycare, waiting rooms, hospitals, schools and the movies. It also meant I was sent home without chemotherapy.

Throughout the process I tested borderline and low for red blood cells or anemia – making me tired, weak and having chest pains. No stairs for me! When I tried to do laundry I was immediately out of breath like

I was having a heart attack. Eventually, I was given three transfusions to bring up my blood count. Again, I was worried about the blood because I was RH Negative and blood type O – and worried the hospital wouldn't have my rare type. Of course, they did have it. I want to thank people who give blood donations – because you're helping someone like me!

About halfway through chemotherapy, I asked my nurse two things. One was about my hair and one was about the ringing in my ears. "Pssst...how come I'm the only one without hair in this joint?" We both smiled and looked down the row of patients sporting every hair-do imaginable. She laughed and said that not everyone loses their hair during chemo and that some of the patients just needed a transfusion and were not there because of something cancer related.

People are so different that I started growing hair three months into chemotherapy treatment (hoping I'm not one of the few who never grows some of their hair back on their head due to full brain radiation), contradicting popular belief. The first of the hair to grow in was just above my cranial scar – it was the only patch that was brown and actually resembled a heart.

By the third month I had grown very itchy on my eyes and knew it meant I was about to lose my eyelashes. I also lost some to most of my hair on my arms, legs and eyebrows. One night I noticed while looking in the mirror that I had hair sprouting from my new sideburns like a Billy-goat! I'll need to start investing in razors, I thought!

I told my nurse I had bouts of ringing in my ears – both ears – a few times a day. I'm so glad I asked about something so trivial because it was actually a big deal. The oncologist mentioned that I should see an ENT (Ears, Nose and Throat) Doctor. The other physician mentioned that Cisplatin is known to cause ringing in the ears, as does full brain Radiation.

Hold onto your horses, though. This is the secret no one dared to tell me about regarding cancer. Early menopause! (Dum; Dum; Duuuum. It's just another thing I learned about cancer that I wished I hadn't; so grateful we had the baby when we did). I had my menses the first two months, but after that it evaporated. The bad news about early menopause is that the low levels of estrogen can lead to osteoporosis, increased risk of colon and ovarian cancer, gum disease, tooth loss and cataracts.

In addition to Cisplatin, I was on a high dose of Navelbine – which was a push drug (pushed right into the IV). The side effects that I experienced were about the same – nausea and vomiting, fatigue, diarrhea and joint pain. The drug didn't seem as bad as the Cisplatin and I rarely vomited.

Shortly after I overcame my virus, I went to the Cancer Care infusion room to have my blood drawn through my forearm. Unfortunately, the one good vein I had for an IV was used in the ER and was black and blue. Two oncology nurses made several attempts to draw my blood, without success.

I was asked to contact Dr. O'Brien, a Surgeon from the hospital that I worked in, to surgically implant a port in my chest. I really didn't want the port because I was afraid and didn't want another surgery, but now I am relieved that I did it. The port connects to a major vein in the upper chest and is accessed every time I have blood-work done which is every time prior to Chemotherapy.

I just had to remember to put Lidocaine on the port up to four hours prior to my blood being drawn or I would feel the needle going into my chest. Also I was told that most people keep the port in for six months after treatment and have it flushed in case blood needs to be taken due to the disease.

That same day I decided to call Dr. O'Brien's office. He asked for a brief consultation with me prior to surgery. On 5/3/13, I went to the Day Surgery department for my port. I was drinking a bottle of water and the nurse's got really upset with me. As it turns out, I was supposed to be completely NPO (no food or drink after midnight). I thought I could have water. I almost didn't have the surgery.

Luckily, one of the nurses didn't think I would be completely out of it during surgery and gave her approval for the surgery to continue. The

Anesthesiologist took me down the hallway in the stretcher for my fourth surgery. He asked if I ever had the medication, Versed. I said, "Yes, I've had plenty of medications."

He gave me half of the meds and put the remainder in the syringe in his pocket. Just prior to us arriving he said, "Do you feel it yet?" I said, "I don't feel anything." He gave me the remainder of the injection. Again, I was intubated. This time I didn't remember the room or anything! The great thing about Versed is that it has amnesic properties.

The port is inserted just below the skin and feels rubbery with three prongs (for the nurse's to access it for blood). For some reason, my one year old son always had a knack at throwing a matchbox car, a book or the remote right onto the port. Finally, I asked the nurse if the port could be damaged. She told me that the port is stitched in and could be turned around if it were hit and that it had happened before. From that point on, I learned to protect the area in front of it.

I don't even remember talking to the doctor after surgery. My husband assured me that I hadn't said anything embarrassing! All went well and I was ready to start Chemotherapy on 5/6/13. I was scheduled to have four cycles (four months) of weekly Chemo with hydration.

Chapter 16

The Start of Chemotherapy

On 5/6/13, I started chemotherapy. The first thing the oncology nurse told me is that my shirt was too high in the neck to gain access to the port. It reminded me how new the process was to me. She kindly asked that I wear a button down shirt for the next time. I heard that the chemotherapy drugs gain strength over time and that I probably wouldn't get sick for a few days, if at all since everyone is different. However, I was given plenty of anti-nausea medications to off-set it.

I looked around. The Infusion Room was one medium sized room with six lounge chairs and a bathroom. The oncology nurses sat directly in front of us and documented their charts on the computers. There were warm blankets available and televisions with headsets overhead. Patients could also read, eat, sleep, do crosswords or nothing at all. There was also food and drink available and curtains between each chair for privacy. I noticed that every person sitting in the chairs was humbled and pleasant.

Each chair had two trays on either side. One side was used for personal belongings while the other tray was for the nurse to place her sterile equipment. Also, an IV pole and vital sign machine stood on either end of the chair. I waited nervously for the nurse to obtain my blood through the new port. All went well and we waited for the results before chemotherapy could begin. About a half hour later, I was told my numbers were good and we could start chemotherapy.

Cisplatin was scheduled every Monday for two weeks for about two and a half hours, along with a push of Navelbine. The remainder of time and the next two days were reserved for hydration since Cisplatin can affect the kidneys. Navelbine was scheduled every Monday for the other two weeks for about an hour and a half. It was a push drug so the nurse connected it to the IV and literally pushed the drug into my blood stream for about ten minutes, followed by hydration.

My mother came up to help and my stepfather dropped her off from Connecticut. She stayed with us for two weeks. When my mom asked if she should come, I said, "I think every girl would want her mom right now." That's all she needed to hear. She was very gracious, refusing our bed, and taking the sofa instead. On the days I had chemo, she dropped me off. She also paid for Joseph to go to daycare for most of the summer.

This was a big discussion in our home. David was dead set against Joseph going to daycare because he was afraid of him catching viruses as he was almost never sick. David also wasn't sure that he trusted caregivers with his son.

However, my first two children started daycare less than six weeks after birth and they were both fine. Yes, they contacted a lot of illness but they socialized earlier. I also trusted that most people wanted to be around children because they liked them; not because they wanted to hurt them. Joseph had been home for almost two years with David and I working opposite schedules. It was time for Joe to make his own friends. I also needed 'me' time. I needed to rest during chemo. I simply couldn't take care of him by myself when I was sick.

Joseph was a handful. He was very active and mischievous – as I've said, I called him Curious George. Not only curious, but fast! I thought he was probably bored being in the house. We made a decision after months, to start him in daycare. Our friends made a schedule so that when my mom went home, they could bring Joseph to daycare, too. We visited the daycare so David could feel comfortable with the caregivers and Joseph could feel comfortable with his surroundings.

I'll never forget it. I laid on the couch nauseous while my Mom called the daycare and asked if they had any openings. They didn't. But after learning about my story, the director said she would move one of the children to another room, opening up a space for Joseph. The next day we visited the daycare.

Shy and timid Joseph actually slid out of David's arms and started playing with the other children and toys. We all watched incredulously. We had to literally pick him up twenty minutes later because he didn't want to leave. It was socially healthy for him.

I, on the other hand, needed to wear a mask whenever I dropped him off of picked him up. And still, both Joseph and I – and David – all were sick for about a month as we contracted almost every virus imaginable – a cough, vomiting and sore throat. And yet, we still thought that daycare was more favorable than Joseph sitting around at home – or running wild at home!

The disappointment came when it was time to do chemo. On three occasions the nurses took my blood and sent me home – I was either Neutropenic (Low white cells) or Anemic (Low red cells). On one occasion I actually cried. I just wanted to get the chemo over with instead of extending it.

Neutropenia is when the fighter cells are so low that the person can pick up any dangerous virus. It can cause vomiting which happened to me more often than not. I had to wear a mask in closed spaces and around my son. Most of the time I started sweating under the mask and had to remove it and take my chances.

Anemia is when the red blood cell count is low. Cisplatin has a reputation of sucking up the red blood cells from the bone marrow, as well as the white blood cells. Anemia can cause chest pains, pale skin, fatigue, shortness of breath and vomiting. It was an intricate balance to stay healthy.

The doctors decided to put me on Neupogin Shots to bring up my white cell count. It was a refrigerated shot that was delivered to my home because it was cheaper to pay for it that way than pay $20 for each shot at the hospital. The only issue wasn't the needle – that didn't hurt at all – it was the serum in the shot that would feel like a bee sting and I would cry. A lot of times Joseph would hold my hand when I had it done. Of course, that would prevent me from crying because I didn't want to scare him.

Depending on my white blood cell levels, I might have to have shots once every three to five days. Most of the time, David gave me my shots. We learned that hard way that the shot could not be given within twenty four hours of chemotherapy; yes, I was sent home again when David forgot and gave me my shot late – within twenty four hours of chemotherapy. He felt horrible. But I don't get upset over such things anymore.

I didn't want Joseph to see me getting sick or falling asleep much of the day due to fatigue. I didn't want him to see me crying. I wanted him to be cheerful and inquisitive. I wanted him to see Brittany and say, "I love you, Butt-Butt" (which is what he called her ever since he could talk – even though he can say, Brittany).

I tried to be strong and have a stiff upper lip. Inevitably, the pain of the cancer would rise to the surface.

Brittany experienced her own pain in her own way. She started to have panic attacks and wondered if some of her symptoms were from cancer. The first time she had a panic attack she was home alone. David was at work, Joseph was at school and I was hooked up to chemotherapy. What a horrible and helpless feeling to not run to your child who is ill.

I had a good friend go to the house and speak with her and bring her to the hospital where I was. I cried. I cried about how I affected every person in and out of our family. I felt guilty for causing everyone pain. I hoped Brittany would be okay. It was good for Brittany to talk about her feelings. We don't communicate enough in our family. Change must happen. We must speak up about things that are troubling us. This is one example of how a negative situation can be turned into something positive.

David had a hard time handling things, too. He was often angry – angry at cancer, I guess. Every day was like a crazy eight ball – you'd never know the message in the window until you shook it up.

Chapter 17

Chemotherapy and Kudos

Most of the time, my nurse was Susan M. and I loved her. I always looked forward to talking with her. Don't get me wrong – the other nurses were great – but my favorite was Susan M. She whisked around the floor like she was on ice skates. I liked just watching her and seeing what a profound professional she was. She knew that I was always cold in the Infusion Room and immediately turned up the heat and put a warm blanket around my shoulders and another over my legs. She pampered me.

Dr. Jackman was great, too. I remember one night I didn't know if we should have a Neupogin shot and I made nine phone calls and couldn't get a hold of anyone. Finally, and in a panic, I called Dr. Jackman at Brigham and Women's Hospital on a Friday night around seven thirty pm. The answering service said he was still in the office and they would contact him. Not two minutes later, he called me.

I said, "I know you probably don't remember me, but my name is Sherry Guarneri." He laughed and said, "Sherry, of course I remember you! We were just talking about you." It made me feel pretty special. I asked him my question about Neupogin but he didn't believe that I needed the shot, anyway. It turned out that I did! Not taking it was the first time my white blood cell count went too low. But I don't think it mattered much at that point. I was grateful that someone was on the other end of the phone. He remembered me.

When I went back to Cancer Care, Dawn heard what happened and sat down to speak with me. She said that a lot of times I wouldn't need the shot because I could go to the hospital after hours and get it done at Brigham's. She gave me a private phone number where I could get a hold of her. I really appreciated her knowledge, sensitivity and kindness.

Chemotherapy was difficult. For the first couple of months I was sick a majority of the time. I couldn't seem to pass a sink without puking in it. I was fatigued and couldn't wait to sleep. When I woke up, I couldn't wait to go back to sleep.

Part of that was depression, even though I was put on an anti-depressant when I was told I had cancer. Sometimes I would try to sing a song and the next moment I would burst out crying. I was overly sensitive. I guess staring at life and death in the face can do that to someone.

I was grateful for all of the support of the hospital, so I picked out a cake for the Special Care Unit – where I used to work, and one for Med Surgery South and Med Surgery North that said 'thank-you' on the top of it. I picked out one very special cake for the ladies and men of the emergency room. In my condition I probably should have been giving out fruit and veggie plates, but if I couldn't have cake, someone else should enjoy it!

About six weeks later, I seemed to suffer from a bout of laryngitis. The longer I spoke in general and through-out the day, the more I struggled to talk. Finally, after about six weeks and the physician's worrying the hoarseness was from GERD (Gastroesophageal Reflux Disease), my bronchoscopy, thrush or allergies, I went to see an Ears, Nose and Throat Specialist (ENT).

Thank God my friend Donna came with me so I could hold her hand for moral support. I was truly frightened to go through a procedure without being unconscious. What I missed more than anything was not being able to sing anymore without my voice cracking. Singing was my thing! I knew every song from the fifties and on and loved everyone from classical to hip hop. My kids have definitely gotten their singing or head bopping from this parent.

Dr. Parker Chamberlin was compassionate and kind as he performed this most routine of exams. But I was nervous. My husband had gone to an ENT and I knew what was about to happen. After taking a brief history, he plunged Lidocaine down each nostril and gave it a moment to set in.

A snake-like light slid down my right nostril at the direction of Dr. Chamberlin. "Swallow, swallow, swallow." It felt really weird, but once it was in, I didn't feel a thing. He checked out my vocal cords, thinking one had been frozen due to the bronchoscopy, but he found nothing of the sort. After removing the tube he shared that he thought perhaps the problem was GERD or a side effect from Cisplatin. We would know for sure in another month once my chemotherapy treatment was finally complete!

Chapter 18

A Word About People

Of course when you're struggling with cancer, life doesn't stop. I lost my health insurance, as did my children (my husband never had any insurance other than dental because his job didn't offer it and I couldn't afford it), unless we wanted to pay for a Cobra policy, after my short term disability ended, which was over a thousand dollars a month (which was about what I made for income). I worried I would never get health insurance again if I switched jobs.

I cried endless tears because I couldn't get prescriptions for my daughter or myself during this overlap. The cobra for insurance was twelve hundred dollars a month! We were told we made 'too much money' for state assistance, but we were just over the poverty line.

One month I got a letter in from Maine Care stating we weren't approved for insurance because my husband and I were both felons! I called them right away and insisted they redo the letter correctly. The response was, "You're making a big deal out of nothing. She just checked the wrong box." Really? No big deal???

It made us angry that we truly needed the help and bought the cheapest groceries at the store and witnessed others who got help because they knew how to work the system and put the most expensive groceries into their cart without thinking twice or because they decided not to work.

I think that a step level program is more efficient to help empower people to help themselves. But for every person who takes advantage of help, it seems that honesty via friends is just as powerful. Big thanks to Lisa, Claims Assistant and Organizational Extraordinaire for helping us through the insurance crunch!

I recall the hours spent trying to get medication for my daughter and shots for myself because my white blood cell count had gone too low. I was told by the pharmacy and by Curascript (for the refrigerated shots) that I needed to get a hold of my insurance company because there was a lapse in coverage over a forty eight hour period.

I was even willing to pay cash – money was no obstacle when it came to our health – but I was ignored and even told the shots were a couple of thousand dollars each. I sat on the couch with the customer service representative on the phone, and cried. My husband grabbed the phone and slipped on a suit of armor. He raised his voice and even swore at the other end of the phone that I was crying on the couch and needed my medications. When he also got nowhere, he lowered his voice and apologized. Somehow and in some way, we got our medication, through the help of our friends.

Our medical bills were piled higher than a Jenga set and left unopened on the counter. Half the time MaineCare said we had insurance; the other half of the time we were told not to pay any bills because we weren't supposed to pay a dime. We were constantly confused and not wanting to ruin our credit - turning in bottles for cash – for stamps, gas, etc. Our cable had been shut off twice and we constantly got nasty grams and phone calls from credit collection companies. Both of our vehicles were illegal for months – due to late registration, vehicle inspections and corrections (i.e. brakes and front tires). And this was all on top of the help that our friends and family were already giving us.

We were proud people. We accepted a lot of the help. We learned to say, "Yes", more than "No". But we still had pride. We had a difficult time staring generosity in the face. So, a lot of the times, people didn't know the stressors that were affecting us. I suppose it's our own fault; but we didn't want to burden people more than what we already did.

I would like to extend a few amazing moments and divine interventions that stopped my heart other than the fact that my cancer was found in time and in the first place.

John, one of the brothers who owns Genuine Auto, cleaned our brakes, gave us an earned inspection sticker and changed two expensive tires for the price of just the parts instead of parts and labor. John changed our lives.

Dr. Pier, who owns Midcoast Dentistry, sent me a heartwarming cards and submitted my dental claims but they were surprising always paid for. Dr. Pier changed our lives.

Meghan, Director of Midcoast Children's Development and our neighbor, who moved people around to make a space for Joseph and for submitting him for a partial scholarship. Meghan, you changed our lives.

Sherrie from Union, you saw me dancing and singing with my baby son in the shopping parking lot. You stopped walking into the store and knocked on my window. You cried when you told me you had survived Thyroid Cancer. You were diagnosed when your son was a year and a half. You went to Brigham's Hospital, too. You gave me a pamphlet for acupuncture and told me it would change my life. I introduced my name as, "Sherry." Your name is, "Sherrie." Sherrie, you changed our lives.

Josh, you were selling photographs you had taken in Boothbay Harbor. You asked if I was a survivor. When I said yes, you called me over and showed me your brain scar from cancer. You were going back into Radiation treatment because it reoccurred. You gave me a beautiful photo of a butterfly – my thank-you cards all had butterfly's on them. You said to keep in touch. Josh, you changed our lives.

Thank-you, Donna (Nah-Nah) for befriending our baby. For your friendship. For bringing over an air-conditioner that we couldn't afford, but couldn't afford not to have with breathing problems in the humidity. Thank-you for filling our tank with gas. Thank-you for scheduling my time.

Thank-you, Tracy (Tah-Tah) for being our financial friend. For hugs and kisses, encouragement and optimism in the line of fire. Thank-you for filling our tank with gas. Thank-you for scheduling our Meal Train. Thank-you for your friendship. Thank-you for your understanding and support. Thank-you for your note-taking.

Thank-you, Sarah (Just Sarah) for being our insurance friend. You gave me rides to and from chemotherapy. You were an RN to my medical problems. You gave us free care and directed us through the messy line of insurance claims.

Thank-you, Jasmine (Just Jas) for being my supportive and funny friend. You gave me rides in the dead of winter to chemotherapy with sleepy eyes and wild hair. You made me laugh when I wanted to cry. You have been my Jade Plant.

Thank-you, David for being who you are. Thank-you for being my friend and husband. Thank-you for holding my hand. Thank-you for your love and support. Thank-you for the untold and private story of us.

Thank-you, Brett, Brittany and Joseph. I love you. Whomever you decide to be.

Thank-you to my extended family especially Mom for being a pit bull with lipstick, for your financial support of Joe's daycare, for inspiring and encouraging me to build upon my strengths into the lady that I have become today.

Thank-you to the spirits alive and departed. There are many more perfect strangers, family and friends that I would like to thank for being my hero…but they are too many to list here. You know who you are.

Chapter 19

Final Exams

In late July, 2013, I had a brain MRI done. A few days later, I had a PET Scan completed. I was more worried about the PET scan due to spread than anything. The morning I was supposed to get back the results of my PET scan, my stomach did the twist and shout. Dawn from Cancer Care told me in seconds that both tests came back negative.

And yet, there was no big sigh of relief. There was just relief. Still, the black cloud hovered. I was cancer-free. I suppose I will never feel complete relief but some relief from being told I'm cancer-free. Every three months; then every six; then every year I will have tests done to see if the cancer spread. I was told that the first two years are the most important. Until then, I can only live and breathe for today.

As of August 20th, I was done with chemotherapy. I ended my relationship with Cancer Care by bringing in a gourmet cake and flowers as a thank-you. There are no words to describe our gratitude that I am alive. Every day that went by, I smiled a little bit bigger; I felt a little bit stronger. The first time I washed the dishes; drove my car; did the laundry – was a milestone – my confidence was finally growing back. I am now a few weeks away from my last appointment with Brigham and Women's Hospital and Dr. Jackman and Dr. Swanson.

In October 2013, I plan on returning to work part time, after my fundraiser in mid-September. I plan on advocating for those who survive – and don't survive – cancer. I have already started. I have written this book to help those have some hope. I have spoken to people about a tennis tournament with donations going to the American Lung and American Cancer Society. I have spoken with the American Red Cross about providing spreadsheets to those attending fundraisers to sign up to donate/volunteer and have investigated ways to do the same for bone marrow donations. I have ordered white and silver cancer pins for our hospital gift shop. I have asked the American Lung Cancer Society to provide literature and brochures regarding lung cancer. I have personally donated money and participated in a 5K run for the American Lung Cancer Society. My work continues.

Chapter 20

Cancer

The fingers of cancer touch every life in one way
or another. This must be why I struggled with survivor's
guilt. I watched CNN every day and was horrified with
each news episode and yet I was addicted to watching it.
People lost limbs and lives but I lived. I cried. I didn't
think I was good enough to live. I hated that I made
people upset or averted their eyes when they saw me. I
went through a period when I cried through
chemotherapy. I wanted the blankets that were wrapped
around my legs to be wrapped around my head for some
privacy. These were my most private moments.

I twisted and turned with insomnia in my bed.
Finally, I sobbed when I spoke with the well-dressed
lady and Cancer Care social worker, Ginny (who also
connected me with a Look Good Feel Good Program

where I received booklets, advice, friendship and $500 worth of fresh make-up!). The bottle lid finally burst off like I shattered a bottle of sparkling water when I spoke with Ginny.

I was still crying when my friend, Sarah, brought me home. Everything disturbing that crossed my mind came up and I didn't even remember what I said to her but I talked nonstop from the hospital to my house. I needed to vent. I needed to cry. I needed to question. I needed sleep…and it was only through venting to the social worker and my friend that I finally got some shut-eye that night.

I survived cancer. Why me? What is my purpose? I have one, or I wouldn't be here. Is it to tell my story? Did I endure the pain to write about how I felt when it happened? Am I strong enough to share my pain with others? Am I the person who has been chosen to advocate for others? That's what I choose to believe. It is what I must believe. I also believe there is a reason why you chose this book. Stop and think. What is your purpose? Are you fulfilling it? Or does God need to send a bolt of lightning to get through to you too, like me?

I recall a long time ago – shortly after the tragedy of September 11th, - in New York City, having a dream in which I was sitting at a table with my spirit guide. I couldn't see his face – just his shirt. He said to me, "What is your purpose?" I thought about it and said, "To help people." He was pleased with my response. When I woke up, I knew that my dream was a divine intervention.

Just like the divine intervention of finding out that I had cancer. The 'knowing' of humming, 'If I Only Had a Brain'. Just like the garden rock that my sister-in-law Katrina gave to me as a birthday present a year before my diagnosis that said, 'Expect a Miracle.' I did. The intervention and insistence of one radiologist for me to get a second Brain MRI with contrast. I trusted his knowledge and intuition. Thank God. Thank you, God.

Conclusion

Today I stand strong. I am strongly rooted into the ground. As strong as that beautiful tree named Shuzie. There are times that I blossom like the summer months. There are times that I am withered and bare like the winter months. There are times that I bend and refuse to break.

I will be here as long as Shuzie is whispering in the wind with her guidance. She directs a path towards advocating; forever changing the lives of all who are affected.

Thank you for sharing my journey with...and beside me

Addendum

On Wednesday, October 19th, I was giddy with delight at the prospect of returning to work. I bought new grey and pink scrubs and fluorescent socks and sneakers. I Facebooked my friends and co-workers with the update and told them I would see them in a couple of hours. I was getting breakfast in the kitchen when my cell phone rang in the living room.

I didn't get to it in time, but listened to the voice mail of my Oncologist asking me to call her about my most recent MRI and PET scans completed in the prior two days. I called back immediately but got voice mail. Not receiving a phone call in an hour and just wanting to hear the words that all was well, I called Cancer Care back and asked to speak with the Oncologist. I said I was fine but my husband was about to vomit.

The Oncologist got on the phone. I will never forget her first words to me. "Sherry, I have a little bit of bad news for you." Oh no, I thought, I'm alone again. I anchored my body against the dining room wall, unclear of how bad the news would be.

"The PET scan looks okay but the MRI with contrast of your brain is showing that the tumor has grown back in your brain. Remember where it grew before?" I said, "Yes." She said, "It's in the same area but arterially and laterally. It looks like it's coming out of the original crevice where Dr. Florman removed the tumor." My cancer was as stubborn as me. Not only did it survive the original craniotomy and two and a half weeks of full brain radiation, but it continued to grow – and in an upwards motion towards the grey matter of my brain.

"What now?" I asked. She continued, "I've been on the phone with both Dr. Florman and Dr. Healey to decide the next steps. Once we have a plan in place, I will call you back." My steadiness turned to tears. My Oncologist said, "Hang in there, Sherry." I tried, I really did. But I was absolutely shocked and devastated this time around.

My husband immediately came home and we hugged. We knew that this could happen but we weren't expecting it so soon. My wise husband said, "This is not a sprint; it's a marathon." I had to agree with him. Maybe the Neurosurgeon just, 'missed a spot.' We waited for another hour and finally got the news. Dr. Healey, the Radiologist from Augusta, suggested direct radiation called an SRS. Stereotactic Radiation Therapy allows a higher dose of radiation to a small focused area in the size of millimeters.

Still not feeling confident with the plan, I contacted Dana Farber and spoke with my primary oncologist. He agreed with the plan and stated an additional craniotomy would be difficult and the next line of therapy would be to try direct radiation – especially since the brain can only be radiated in one place per lifetime. First I had the whole brain radiation, which was apparently not strong enough, as Dr. Healey explained. Now we would try two weeks' worth of full brain radiation into one large gamma ray of direct radiation.

He explained during our initial meeting that although the brain MRI showed a shadow, it was initially thought to be 'residual' from the first surgery. In actuality, it was the brain tumor growing back.

First, I would be fit for two masks in Augusta. One mask would be like a cast behind my head. The second mask would be fitting to the front of my face and screwed down around my head. My hands would remain still, holding securely to poles on either end of my hips. Fitting me with the masks would take the most time – a couple of hours. The name of the game was Precision. The mathematical equation needed to be precise which is why they used a team, including a Physics Doctor. The second appointment was the actual direct radiation, on Friday October 29th, 2013.

The actual radiation only took a few minutes and I took two Ativan prior to my appointment so I didn't panic with the masks. The actual radiation only lasted about five minutes and I think I fell asleep during some of it. The only difference I noticed at first was the worst metal taste in my mouth when I woke up a few times during the night.

The after effects were more prevalent. In the days to come I had front and back headaches – not bad enough for me to warrant a phone call at first – some wobbles into the walls and backwards, my usual lack of some words (calling my Dexamethasone pill a Dexatrim pill instead) and I should mention after a few days and by taking Dexamethasone for brain swelling as prescribed by my doctors, the headaches immediately disappeared.

I was afraid to call the doctor at first because of my history of anxiety; but they took my concerns as seriously as I and it worked. They listened to me. It's important to share your greatest fears and indiscretions.

Unfortunately, it takes six to eight weeks for the brain tumor to stop multiplying and vacate the area. Therefore, I won't know if the direct radiation worked until then. It's a long ways to wait...until after the holidays. If Plan A does not work, Plan B is to do a second craniotomy in Boston. We are willing to try anything; do anything; go anywhere.

Between my appointments, I knew I wanted to pray the rosary and share the despair that had been placed upon my heart. The day after hearing the bad news, I drove myself to three chapels after I dropped off my son at childcare. The first was a Catholic church. A man was cooking in the back; took one look at my tear streamed face and said, "I sure wish I was a priest right now." He compassionately told me to check another church, as the doors were locked.

I drove to the second church. The doors were locked. I drove twenty minutes to another church…and Episcopal Church…and set off the alarms. It was another divine intervention, like God screaming, "This is an emergency!" The Deacon rushed over from across the street to shut off the alarm and met me. She took me into another room and listened to my long story with great compassion. I felt better once I could get the burden off of my soul.

She found me a set of rosary beads and called me the following morning to pick them up. It was after then and when we met the priest – who was also a cancer survivor – that we decided we would have our son Joseph christened there. What a wonderful set of circumstances. Thank you, God. I did the Radiation with a blue pouch on my stomach full of rosary beads, a pin that said, "Mom" from the Deacon Rosalee (like Rosary), a blinged out cancer survivor pin and my cross that said, "Faith Can Move Mountains."

The next Monday, after Radiation, I drove myself to the Social Security Office. They were actually wonderful and were able to approve myself and my kids for Social Security Disability because I was at Stage IV. I never even knew – or thought – that I could qualify for that. Although wonderful, again it was painful and I cried when it was done and over with.

Again, as I sat in the waiting room and looked around I saw many people who would probably qualify but didn't need to. I also tried to get heating assistance, but was told that since we were $138 over the poverty level, we couldn't be approved. We were also co-paying for an insurance claim through David's company that he signed almost six weeks to the day prior when I found out I had cancer. Washington National said, "So sorry; but you are a few weeks into the probationary period so we won't be paying you or reimbursing you for both of your hospital claims for cancer."

I could feel the anger rise again; but I knew inside I was on my journey; they were on theirs. God would take care of us. Anger can only eat your soul. Every night I still pray for my life; every morning I still pray for the joy of breathing. Until we know different, I will be working with my local church and volunteering as much as I can. In January, a new year may bring new doors to open. I am somewhat reserved yet hopeful again.

The End?

Printed in Great Britain
by Amazon

28129239R20108